MW00658642

Chinese Nutrition Therapy

Dietetics in Traditional Chinese Medicine (TCM)

Joerg Kastner, MD, LAc
Private Practice
Wessling, Germany

2nd edition

Thieme
Stuttgart · New York

Library of Congress Cataloging-in-Publication Data

Kastner, Jörg, 1963-
[Propädeutik der chinesischen Diätetik. English]
Chinese nutrition therapy : dietetics in traditional Chinese medicine (TCM) / Joerg Kastner. -- 2nd ed.
p. ; cm.
Authorized and revised translation of the 2nd German edition published and copyrighted 2003 by Georg Thieme Verlag, Stuttgart, Germany.
Includes bibliographical references and index.
ISBN 978-3-13-130962-4 (alk. paper)
1. Dietetics. 2. Medicine, Chinese. 3. Diet therapy.
4. Nutrition.
I. Title. [DNLM: 1. Nutrition Therapy--methods. 2. Diet.
3. Medicine, Chinese Traditional. WB 400 K192p 2009a]
RM217.K3313 2009
613.2--dc22
2008043605

This book is an authorized and revised translation of the 2nd German edition published and copyrighted 2003 by Hippokrates Verlag, Stuttgart, Germany. Title of the German edition: Propädeutik der Chinesischen Diätetik.

Original translator: Johanna Cummings-Pertl, Ukiah, CA, USA
Updated new edition: Sabine Wilms, PhD, Ranchos de Taos, NM, USA

Joerg Kastner, MD, LAc
www.zentrum-ganzheitsmedizin.de
kastner@zentrum-ganzheitsmedizin.de

Rüdigerstrasse 14, 70469 Stuttgart, Germany
http://www.thieme.de
Thieme New York, 333 Seventh Avenue,
New York, NY 10001, USA
http://www.thieme.com

Cover design: Thieme Publishing Group
Typesetting by Fotosatz Sauter GmbH, Donzdorf, Germany
Printed in Germany by CPI Books

ISBN 978-3-13-130962-4 4 5

Contents

"Let food be your medicine
and medicine be your food."

Hippocrates, ca. 460–ca. 370 BC

About this Book

The concepts of Chinese nutrition, or the effects of food on our health, have a 3000-year tradition in China. Records dating back as far as the third century BC state that there was little difference between the application of foods and that of medicine. Recipes for foods were often similar to those for medicines.

A quote by a famous fourteenth-century physician describes the role of Chinese nutrition within Traditional Chinese Medicine (TCM): *"Doctors first have to find the cause for an illness and determine which disharmony prevails. To balance this disharmony,* ***the first and foremost*** *measure is appropriate diet. It is not until this measure bears no results that one should use medicines."*

Chinese nutritional therapy is closely related to acupuncture and medicinal plant medicine and follows the same diagnostic principles. It focuses on the qualitative effects of foods on the body. The term "*qi*," which has many meanings in Chinese, including *life force* or *life energy*, is of vital significance in this context. Health is an expression of balanced *qi*; disease occurs when *qi* is unbalanced. The body extracts and absorbs *qi* from food. Foods, therefore, are mild therapeutic agents that help the body stay balanced, or bring it back into balance. Food classification follows the same criteria used for Chinese medicinal herbs: thermal nature, flavor, organ network, and direction of energy flow.

Chinese culture reflects an awareness of the healing qualities of food as a kind of folk wisdom, even today. Food and health are favorite topics of conversation. "Did you eat well today?" replaces "Hello" as a popular greeting. What we regard as complicated is practiced on a daily basis in China, for example, the simple balancing of hot and cold: Cold weather is balanced by eating foods that have a warming effect on the body, such as ginger tea, garlic, fennel, oats, lamb, salmon, etc. Hot weather is balanced by eating cooling foods such as raw fruit and vegetables, salads or, barley.

This knowledge of the healing qualities of food was practiced and treasured in our own culture until recently, but has gotten lost in the trend toward "fast food." Similar connections between food and medicine have been made since antiquity. Hippocrates recommended "*Let food be your medicine and medicine be your food.*" Hildegard von Bingen, the eleventh-century German visionary naturalist and healer, used foods for healing by devising energetic classifications that are surprisingly similar to Chinese food classifications. Even the original meaning of the word "dietetics," drawn from the Greek "diaita"—"life care" or "art of living"—shows the comprehensive meaning of diet as supporting life.

Western nutritional therapy, a relatively young science, applies primarily quantitative criteria to food. It classifies food by nutrients such as carbohydrates, protein, fat, vitamins, trace elements, and minerals. For diabetes, for example, it prescribes a quantitative diet that measures the glycemic index of foods. However, there is increasing interest in the qualitative aspects of foods in the Western world, in part due to the rapid increase of food-related illnesses and the observation that people can react very differently and very strongly to the same food. Like acupuncture and medicinal plant therapy, Chinese nutritional therapy can offer valuable perspectives in this context.

Current Western scientific methods are not yet able to offer plausible explanations for the concept of energetics in Chinese nutrition. This difficulty in dealing with unfamiliar concepts starts with the term *qi*, which is viewed with intellectual skepticism in the West. *Qi*, however, can be experienced through the practice of *qi gong* (a healing art that combines movement and meditation).

With this book, I would like to awaken the curiosity in my readers that has always been the spark for moving forward and making progress. Chinese nutrition is a great—and delicious—method for taking a closer look at what we eat and for looking beyond what we know and are used to. It challenges us to practical experimentation, because only those who put theory into practice by cooking will profit—in body and soul!

I am pleased with the positive response *Chinese Nutrition Therapy* has enjoyed in the English-speaking world, as a result of which a second edition has become necessary after only a short time. I would like to use this opportunity to integrate two subjects that seem highly significant in daily clinical practice: overweight and the increasing number of patients who seek my medical advice for the symptoms of physical and/or emotional fatique and exhaustion, to the point of burnout. For these problems, Chinese dietetics has proven extremely helpful and offers excellent options for self-help. I welcome all suggestions, advice, and reports of my readers' experiences, and hope that those of you who have allowed my book to inspire you in your therapeutic or culinary activities meet with success and accomplish your goals!

Fall 2008 *Joerg Kastner, MD, LAc*

Acknowledgements

A heartfelt "thank you" to my parents, who gave me the freedom to walk uncommon paths, and to my teachers, who showed me the way. My gratitude also goes out to my patients, who time and time again have proven to me how consistent integration of Chinese nutrition into our daily diet helps overcome illness and creates health. I am also grateful to all the people who have attended my seminars, for their willingness to be inspired by this initially rather unfamiliar body of thought and to practice its principles in their own life and with their patients. I especially thank my wife, Ulrike, who has stood by me and supported me all the way and who demonstrates to me continually the culinary, sensual pleasures of Chinese nutrition. A big "thank you" also goes out to my editor Angelika-M. Findgott for providing such valuable guidance and showing so much editorial patience, and to Johanna Cummings-Pertl for her meticulous editing of the English translation of this book, and for offering many suggestions for improvements. Together, they made the U.S. edition of this book even better than the German original. I would also like to thank Anne Lamparter for her attentive project management of the second edition and Sabine Wilms for her excellent translation of the new text parts.

Structure and Use of this Book

The first chapter of this book, "Introduction to the Basic Principles of Traditional Chinese Medicine and Chinese Dietetics," introduces Chinese nutrition theory using practical examples. Chapters 2 and 3 introduce Chinese dietetics in practice. Chapter 2 covers key dietary concepts such as healthy eating habits and eating in harmony with seasonal and constitutional factors. Chapter 3 outlines nutritional therapy for the most important pathological processes and provides an overview and orientation framework for symptoms and diagnosis.

Chapter 4, "Food Classification," is based on a variety of source texts and applies their concepts to the most common "Western" foods. Here you will find detailed information about the nature and use of foods and food groups in nutritional therapy. In case of contradictions between the authors regarding classification, I endeavored to classify foods according to my own clinical experience.

The clinical examples in Chapter 5, "Analogy of Western Diagnoses with Syndromes in Traditional Chinese Medicine (TCM)," intend to establish a bridge to Chinese syndrome diagnosis. By their very nature, these offer abridged and incomplete introductions to a very large field of knowledge. They are designed to encourage Western practitioners to combine Western with Eastern thinking. Lay readers are advised that for disorders such as hypertension, asthma, Crohn disease, etc., any therapeutic measure should always be discussed with the treating physician and should be harmonized with Western methods of treatment. My practice, however, has proven to me repeatedly that Chinese nutrition is an excellent complement to Western treatments and also offers outstanding synergies with other naturopathic therapies.

In this book, I have consciously avoided the use of Chinese medicinal plants in recipes. While commonly used in China, Chinese herbal therapy requires many years of experience and a high level of education on the part of the practitioner, as well as reliable quality control of the preparations used.

For the reader in a hurry, Chapter 6 provides charts of the most commonly used foods grouped by organ network. "Foods from A to Z" offers a quick guide to the key characteristics of the most common foods.

The glossary in Chapter 7 provides definitions of the English terms most frequently used in this book and lists their Chinese translations. The terminology used in this book is based on "A Practical Dictionary of Chinese Medicine" by Nigel Wiseman and Feng Ye (Paradigm Publications, 1998, 2nd edition). Thieme International, in choosing this dictionary as its standard, recognizes the monumental contributions that Nigel Wiseman and Feng Ye have made to the standardization of TCM terminology in the English-speaking world. For more information on terminology, see Chapter 7.

△ *Yang*

▽ *Yin*

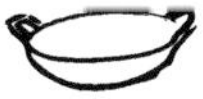 Nutritional therapy

 Recommended foods

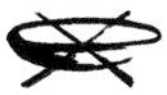 Foods to avoid

 Recipes, dietary recommendations

Basic Recipes:
Congee, page 117
Medicinal wines, page 160
Grains, page 39

激 Acupuncture therapy
Moxibustion

1 Theory

A Introduction to the Basic Principles of Traditional Chinese Medicine and Chinese Dietetics

Yin and *Yang*

The basic principles of Traditional Chinese Medicine (TCM) are rooted in the Taoist philosophy of *yin* and *yang*. These two polar opposites organize and explain the ongoing process of natural change and transformation in the universe.

According to ancient lore, *yang* marks the sunny side and *yin* the shady side of a hill. In the theory of *yin* and *yang*, all things and phenomena of the cosmos contain these two complementary aspects. The traditional Taoist symbol for completeness and harmony is the merging monad of *yin* and *yang*.

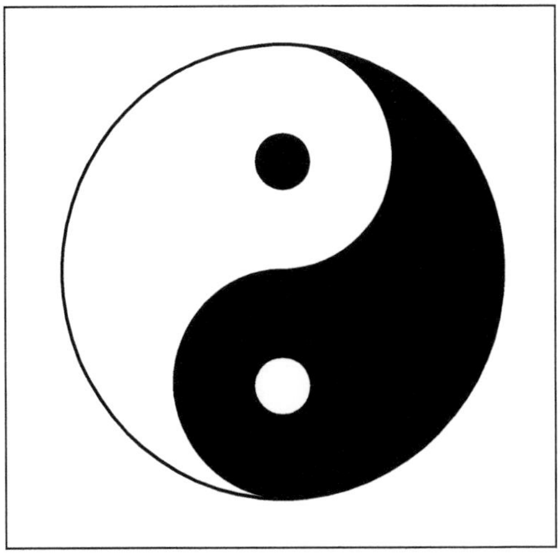

Fig. 1.1 **Monad**

The standard of TCM, the *Huang Di Nei Jing*, "The Yellow Emperor's Classic of Medicine," dates as far back as 500–300 BC. This 18-volume classic work has two parts, *Ling Shu* and *Su We*. The *Su Wen* explains the theoretical foundations of TCM in the form of a dialogue between the legendary Yellow Emperor *Huan Di* and his personal physician *Shi Po*.

The *Ling Shu*, the practical part of the *Nei Jing*, reports on therapies and their uses in TCM: acupuncture, moxibustion, nutritional therapy, and the use of medicinal herbs.

TCM is rooted in the Taoist worldview employed by physicians and philosophers for centuries as a guide for viewing and interpreting natural phenomena.

Tao means harmony–destination–way, the "all-in-one," the origin of the world. The teachings of Taoism are based on the work *Tao te King* (*Tao te Ching*), "The Book of the Way and of Virtue," by the famous Chinese scholar *Lao Tse* (600 BC).

Guided by the Taoist perspective, "natural scientists" took the findings of these observations of nature and applied them to humans. They regarded the human being as a natural being, a part of nature, subject to and dependent on nature's processes.

The main principle of Tao is represented by the two polarities *yin* and *yang*, which, according to Taoist belief, mirror all phenomena in the universe.

In Nature

Yin	Yang
Moon	Sun
Shadow/night	Light/day
Dark	Light
Passive	Active
Water	Fire
Down	Up
Structure	Function
Right	Left
Cold	Hot
Plant-based foods	Animal-based foods
Heaven	Earth
Autumn, winter	Spring, summer
Relative stasis	Evident motion
Heavy	Light

In People

Yin	Yang
Woman	Man
Right	Left
Receptive	Creative
Stomach, front	Back, rear
From waist down	From waist up
Body interior	Body surface
Viscera (storage organs) zang (heart)	Bowels (hollow organs) fu (stomach)
Organ structure	Organ function
Blood, body fluids	Qi, life energy
Bones/organs/ sinews	Skin/muscles/ body hair
Viscera	Bowels
Gu qi (drum qi)	Defense qi (wei qi)
Controlling vessel (ren mai)	Governing vessel (du mai)

In Diagnostics

Yin	Yang
Quiet voice	Loud voice
Talks little	Talks a lot
Pale face	Red face
Shivering, sensation of cold	Warm, sensation of heat
Likes warmth	Likes cold
Slow, reticent movements	Fast, strong movements
Passive, insidious onset of illness	Active, acute onset of illness
Chronic illness	Acute illness
Urine: clear, frequent	Urine: Dark, concentrated
Tongue: pale, white fur	Tongue: Red, yellow fur
Pulse: Slow, weak	Pulse: Rapid, replete

In Diagnostics and Therapy

Yin	Yang
Vacuity, interior, cold symptoms	Repletion, exterior, heat symptoms
Inadequate circulation	Blood repletion
Hypofunction (underfunction)	Hyperfunction (overfunction)
Flaccid muscles	Tense muscles
Depression disorders	States of agitation
Low blood pressure (hypotension)	High blood pressure (hypertension)
Dull pain	Sharp pain
Cool	Warm
Beta-blockers	Caffeine
Cool packs	Fango (hot packs)
Pulse: Slow, deep, rough, vacuous, fine	Pulse: Rapid, floating, slippery, replete, large, surging

In Chinese Nutrition

Yin	Yang
Tropical fruit	Meat
Dairy products	Acrid spices
Seaweed	Shrimp
Orange juice	Coffee
Peppermint tea	Fennel tea
Wheat	Oats
Soy sauce	Tabasco
Wheat beer	Anise schnapps
Steamed foods	Grilled foods

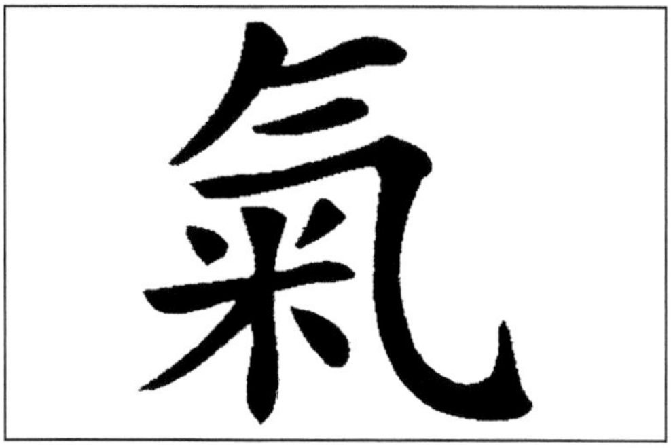

The Symbol for ***Qi***

The Chinese symbol for *qi* is formed by two elements. One element means "air," "breath," "steam"; the other element means "rice," "grains." This character illustrates how something can be both immaterial and material, in accordance with the Taoist principle of *yin* and *yang*.

The energy field between the poles of *yin* and *yang* gives rise to the universal primal force *qi*. According to ancient Chinese belief, vital—or life force—*qi* (*sheng qi*) is the primary source of all living processes in the cosmos.

The concept and meaning of *qi* is only partially translatable into Western languages. Hindus and Yogis use the term "prana" to reflect similar ideas about all-permeating life energy. The ancient Greek term "pneuma" describes a similar concept. Coursing vital *qi*, as an energetic unit, is an essential element in the various treatment modalities of TCM, such as acupuncture, moxibustion, dietetics, medicinal herb therapy, and *qi gong*.

Imbalances of *qi* can take the form of **vacuity** or **repletion**. The term "vacuity" comes from the Chinese "*xu*" (vacuous, empty, lacking, weak). Its opposite is "repletion, " which comes from the Chinese "*shi.* " Vacuity and repletion can be present in varying degrees, from slight to complete (see "Glossary," p. 251, for more details).

Acupuncturists will use needles to modulate strength and speed of *qi* flowing in the channels and to disperse stagnation. *Qi* vacuity can be balanced with foods rich in *qi*, or by strengthening a weakened body with Chinese medicinal herbs.

Therapeutic Principles of TCM

Four basic aspects of interaction between *yin* and *yang* enable practitioners to gain insight into the main processes for development and treatment of diseases. This fundamental understanding of TCM is a requirement for sound diagnoses and effective therapy.

The Four Basic Interactions of *Yin* and *Yang*

1 *Yin* and *yang* are opposites

2 *Yin* and *yang* are divisible but inseparable (*yin yang ke fen er bu ke li*)

3. *Yin* and *yang* are rooted in each other (*yin yang hu gen*)

4 *Yin* and *yang* counterbalance each other (*yin yang zhi yue*)

5 *Yin* and *yang* mutually transform each other

All therapy principles in TCM intend to either retain or reestablish the balance of *yin* and *yang*. Complete balance of *yin* and *yang* means perfect health; imbalance or disharmony between the two poles signifies illness.

Yin And *Yang* are Opposites

Yin and *yang* describe the fundamental properties of two opposites inherent in every object or phenomena in the universe.
These two opposites do not appear, however, to exist in an absolute or static state, for example, light–dark, slow–fast, heaven–earth.

Yin And *Yang* are Divisible but Inseparable (*Yin Yang Ke Fen Er Bu Ke Li*)

Yin And *Yang* are Rooted in Each Other (*Yin Yang Hu Gen*)

The mutual dependency of *yin* and *yang* is essential to understanding *yin* and *yang*. *Yang* cannot exist without *yin* and vice versa.
The *Nei Jjing* states:

"Yin is the root of yang, and yang is the root of yin; no yin can be without yang, and no yang can be without yin."

Yin and *yang* are always interconnected, depend on each other, and conduct an ongoing exchange with each other. Neither of the polarities is ever static. Harmonious unity requires balancing both poles in relationship to each other. They exist in a dynamic, interwoven interplay, similar to the interchange of night and day. For example, activity–rest, above–below, energy–matter, man–woman.

Yin And *Yang* Counterbalance Each Other (*Yin Yang Zhi Yue*)

As is their nature, *yin* and *yang* strive to retain a lasting dynamic balance.
An imbalance in one of the two opposite poles invariably influences the other pole, which changes the relationship of the poles to each other. With *yang* surplus, *yin* gets reduced or consumed. For example, high fever (*yang* repletion) results in a weakening of the body (reduced *yin*) through intense sweating. There are four basic forms of imbalance, which according to TCM explain essential physiological and pathophysiological processes.

Yin repletion with relative *yang* vacuity
→ repletion condition
Yang repletion with relative *yin* vacuity
→ repletion condition
Yin vacuity with relative *yang* repletion
→ vacuity condition
Yang vacuity with relative *yin* repletion
→ vacuity condition

Yin And *Yang* Mutually Transform Each Other

Because *yin* and *yang* create each other, they are always supporting, repairing, and transforming into each other. For example, inhalation is followed by exhalation, and activity is followed by rest.

Even in their seemingly most stable form, *yin* and *yang* are undergoing constant change. This process starts at a specific stage of development. It takes quantitative changes and turns them into qualitative transformations.

The *Nei Jing* states:

"There has to be rest following extensive movement; extreme yang turns into yin."

One example is children at a party: The later it gets, the more excited and noisy they get—their *yang* condition is kept artificially high to suppress their desire for *yin* (sleep)—until it comes to a sudden breakdown, namely *yang* has turned into *yin*. Other examples are life–death, high fever–sudden drop in temperature (shock, blood centralization, cold extremities).

The four basic TCM therapy strategies reflect these fundamental interactions between *yin* and *yang*:

Supplementing *yang*
Supplementing *yin*
Draining *yang* repletion
Draining *yin* repletion

The Five Phases (*Wu Xing*)

The theory of the five phases came into being in the 4th century BC. With its help, *Tsu Yen* (350–270 BC) and his students tried to demystify nature and create an intellectual, rational, self-contained theoretical system.
A Western analogy to this model is the theories shaping Greek antiquity marked by Aristotle.
The Taoist model of the five phases (or elements) is an extension of the concept of *yin* and *yang* developed earlier. It relates the entire spiritual, emotional, material, and energetic phenomena of the universe to five basic phases (earth, metal, water, wood, and fire).
These five phases (or elements) represent natural phenomena that were applied to human beings by the Confucian school:

The Five Phases

Earth	Fertility, ripening, harvest, inner core (center), stability (being grounded), sweet flavor
Metal	Reflection, change, death, acrid flavor
Water	Flow, clarity, cold, birth, salty flavor
Wood	Growth, bending, childhood, expansion, sour flavor
Fire	Heat, flare-up, upbearing, bitter flavor

These phases do not exist in isolation from each other, but influence each other in a constant, dynamic interaction.
With the **engendering** (or feeding) cycle (*xiang sheng*, "mother–child–rule") the phases can nurture each other, for example, water "feeds" wood and makes it grow. Wood nourishes fire and turns into ashes (earth).
The **restraining cycle** (*xiang ke*) keeps the phases in check when one of them grows too powerful. For example, fire controls metal, meaning it melts it. When the restraining cycle breaks down, the resulting disharmony can be viewed in terms of "rebellion" or "overwhelming."
The engendering and restraining cycles reflect harmonious courses of events, whereas the **overwhelming cycle** (*xiang cheng*) and the **rebellion cycle** (*xiang wu*) represent disharmonious events.
The overwhelming cycle is an abnormal exaggeration of the restraining cycle, where one of the phases is weakened, causing the phase that under normal circumstances would restrain it to invade and weaken it further. The rebellion cycle is a reversal of the restraining relationship, where one of the five phases is disproportionately strong and rebels against the phase that should normally restrain it (Wiseman).
For the TCM practitioner, the five phases, in association with their controlling cycles, provide an interesting tool for explaining tendencies and relationships of clinical processes and for finding the right treatment.
The concept of five phases plays an important role in classifying foods and Chinese medicinal herbs.

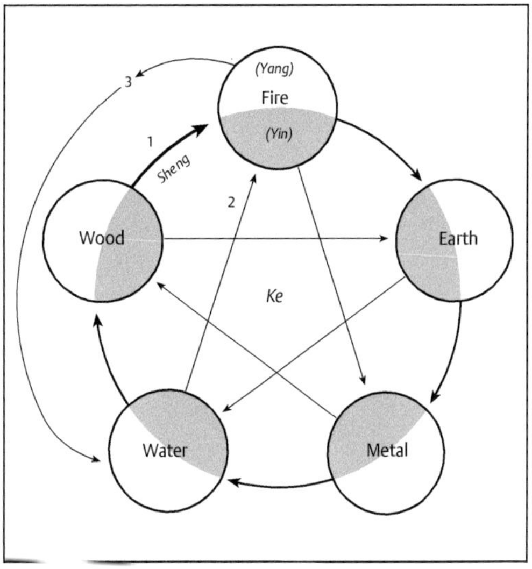

The Five Phases
1 = Engendering *(sheng)* cycle
2 = Restraining *(ke)* cycle
3 = Rebellion *(wu)* cycle

The Five Basic Substances

In TCM, the term "substance" is relative, as it does not contain any determination about matter or energy. This concept builds on an understanding of *yin* and *yang* based on *qi*, which can manifest in different ways, from a total absence of substance for example as spirit/consciousness (*shen*), to material forms, for example as body fluids (blood or other body fluids).

The Five Basic Substances

- Life force—*qi*
- Congenital essence—*jing*
- Blood—*xue*
- Spirit—*shen*
- Body fluids—*jin ye*

For the TCM practitioner, knowledge about and formation of the five basic substances is very important. They are the key parameters addressed by TCM therapy.

Nutritional and herbal therapies are especially valuable for influencing the formation, regulation, and consumption of these basic substances. Attempting to compensate for a deficiency of these substances with acupuncture alone would be a time-consuming process and an ineffective, unsuccessful therapy concept.

Effective therapy, for example in case of blood vacuity (symptom: insomnia), should supplement acupuncture treatment with dietary measures and, if needed, herbal therapy, to promote fast recovery of the patient (e.g., blood-building foods, such as chicken or beef).

Continuous supplementation and regeneration of *qi*, blood, and body fluids is one of the most important tasks of Chinese dietetics.

Life Force—*Qi*

As stated earlier, the term *qi* is usually translated as "energy" or "life force," but the meaning of the term in Chinese is much broader and encompasses aspects that are difficult to translate into Western languages.

In TCM, the vital life force *qi*, source of all life processes in the universe, arises from the energy field between the polarities of *yin* and *yang*.

The Four Basic Forms of *Qi*

- Original *qi* (*yuan qi*)
- *Gu qi* (Wiseman: drum *qi*; synonym: food *qi*, grain *qi*)
- Ancestral *qi* (*zong qi*)
- True qi (zhen qi)

Function

Qi has a variety of functions. *Qi* is the source of all movement in the cosmos. In a medical sense, *qi* is the basic substance of all functions and processes in the human body and the moving force for all life processes. *Qi* warms and protects the body (*wei qi* = defense) and is responsible for growth and development, and for mental and physical activities. *Qi* (*zhen qi*) flows through the channels of the body. Each organ has its own *qi*, which controls the organ's function.

Dysfunction

Qi Vacuity (*Qi Xu*)

Symptoms

General physical weakness, pale complexion, chronic fatigue, loss of appetite, mild sweating, lowered resistance, shortness of breath, quiet voice.

Tongue: Swollen, pale
Pulse: Weak

Nutritional Therapy

Strengthen *qi* with oats, nuts, seeds, warming types of meat and fish (beef, lamb, salmon, trout).

Qi Stagnation (*Qi Zhi*)

Obstruction of *qi* coursing in the bowels and viscera (*zang fu*), channels, or the entire body.

Symptoms

Feeling of pressure, tightness, or oppression; strong, dull, pressing pain; pain in the area of the *qi* coursing disorder (e.g., *qi* blockage in channels), often pain increase with pressure, sometimes with varying intensity and localization of pain. For example, liver *qi* stagnation, tension headaches, rib-side pain.

Tongue: Bluish coloring, prominent lingual veins

Pulse: Tight

Nutritional Therapy

Disperse stagnation with acrid flavors: pepper, chili, high-proof alcohol, Chinese leeks (garlic chives), green onions, fennel, garlic, vinegar, coriander, chili.

Qi Counterflow (*Qi Ni*)

Qi counterflow (a.k.a rebellious or reverse *qi*) is a pathological change of direction of normal *qi* flow.

Symptoms

Nausea and vomiting, hiccoughs, cough, asthma.

Nutritional Therapy

Downbear *qi* with almonds, salt, celery, green tea.

Congenital Essence—*Jing*

The Chinese character for essence means "seed," The classic *Su Wen* states:

"Jing is the origin of the body."

According to TCM, this extremely valuable substance forms the foundation for all physical and mental development. *Jing* is stored in the kidneys; it has no equivalent in Western medicine.

The Two Sources of *Jing*:

- Congenital (constitution) *jing* (prenatal, inherited *jing*) (*xian tian zhi jing*):
  Congenital *jing* is created at conception from parental *jing* (inherited energy, innate energy). It is irrevocably fixed and cannot be replaced or regenerated. This *jing* corresponds to inherited constitution in the Western view.
- Acquired constitution *jing* (*hou tian zhi jing*):
  This *jing* is created by the stomach and spleen after birth from extracted and clear elements of ingested foods and beverages. Acquired *jing* supplements congenital *jing*.

Function

Practitioners of TCM view the amount of *jing* as determining one's quality of life and life expectancy. Since *jing*, as already discussed, cannot be regenerated, it forms a sort of "inner energy clock" which determines our individual life span. Once this "inner energy clock" runs out, the person dies. Understandably, TCM puts great emphasis on the preservation and the careful treatment of *jing*.
Chinese nutritional therapy, as well as many other areas of Asian philosophies, address this important aspect, for example in *qi gong* or tantra.
The quality of *jing* is the foundation for prenatal development of the body. Postpartum, *jing* influences physical and mental growth and is responsible for the body's reproductive strength.

Dysfunction

Poor constitution, premature aging, deformities, sexual disorders such as sterility and infertility.

Nutritional Therapy

Protecting *jing* with a regular diet of healthy and highly nutritious foods and a balanced lifestyle. Supplementing *jing* through dietary measures is not possible.

Blood—*Xue*

Traditionally, blood is viewed as a dense and material form of *qi*. It develops from the essence of food fluids that are extracted by stomach and spleen. The kidneys also contribute to the formation of blood. New *gu qi* obtained from food is transformed via the lung and subsequently connected with ancestral *qi* (*zong qi*). It is then distributed to the entire body by the viscera (*zang* organ) heart.
Blood and *qi* are closely connected.
The *Su Wen* states:

> *"Qi rides on the blood" and further, "Blood is the mother of qi."*

Another passage reads:

> *"When blood and qi develop disharmony, a hundred illnesses can form."*

Function

The most important purpose of blood is to nourish and moisten the body, especially the eyes, skin, hair, muscles, and sinews.
Chinese medicine makes an important connection between the material aspect of blood and immaterial consciousness: "*Blood forms the bed for shen (spirit).*"
Blood, with its *yin* aspect as material basis, is responsible for anchoring the *yang* aspect (spirit or *shen*) within. Blood contains mostly *yin*, but also some *yang*. The spirit is about 98% *yang*, but in Chinese thinking, needs "a little *yin* at night to be able to rest"—this is provided by blood (*xue*). If there is not enough blood, the spirit cannot rest and the result is sleeplessness.
Blood vacuity therefore often displays not only as physical weakness, but also as mental symptoms such as restlessness, forgetfulness, and insomnia.

Dysfunction

Blood Vacuity (*Xue Xu*)

Symptoms
Dull, pale complexion; pale lips, anemia, fatigue, disturbed vision, memory problems, restlessness, insomnia, mental instability.
Tongue: Pale, thin
Pulse: Fine, rough

Nutritional Therapy
Strengthen blood with bass, eel, octopus (squid, cuttlefish), chicken, beef, liver, chicken egg.

Blood Stasis (*Xue Yu*)

Symptoms
Bright, sharp, firmly localized pain, swelling, possibly discoloration of influenced region, purple lips.
Tongue: Dark red, bluish red
Pulse: Tight

Nutritional Therapy
Disperse blood stasis with Chinese leek, venison (deer), vinegar, alcohol.

Blood Heat (*Xue Re*)

Symptoms
Heat sensation, restlessness, dry mouth, skin disorders with red efflorescence, skin itching, bright red bleeding, hypermenorrhea.
Tongue: Red, raised dots
Pulse: Rapid

Nutritional Therapy
Clear blood heat with mung beans, tomatoes, wheat, celery stalks, dandelion, spinach.

Spirit—*Shen*

In TCM, spirit (*shen*) encompasses the mental, psychological, emotional, and spiritual aspects of a person and is expressed in the person's consciousness and personality. Spirit is closely connected with heart, *jing*, blood, and *qi*. These material connections exemplify the unity that mind and body form in TCM. Good spirit shows in the face: it provides a radiant expression and eyes that are alert and clear.

Function

Spirit hosts: Consciousness, thought, memory, sleep, emotions, spirituality, and psyche.
Each viscera (*zang* organ) is accompanied by a psychological–mental aspect:

- **Spirit** soul (*shen*): Heart, consciousness, thought
- **Ethereal** soul (*hun*): Liver, vigor, creativity
- **Corporeal** soul (*po*, body–soul): Lung, instinct, intuition
- **Mind** (*zhi*): Kidney, willpower, character
- **Thought** (*si*): Spleen/pancreas, analytical thinking, memory

Dysfunction

Psychological and mental disorders, insomnia.

Nutritional Therapy
Soothe the spirit, for example with wheat (stabilizes spirit); when agitated, avoid acrid flavor.

Body Fluids—*Jin Ye*

Jin ye incorporates all body fluids. They are extracted by the spleen/pancreas from food and beverages. Body fluids include tears, synovial (joint) fluids, sweat, digestive juices, urine, etc.

Function

TCM distinguishes between two types of body fluid by meaning and function:

Liquid (*Jin*)

Clear, light, thin element; more *yang*; circulates mostly on body surface; keeps skin, hair, ears, eyes, mouth, nose, genitals, and other orifices and muscles moist.

Humors (*Ye*)

Turbid, heavy, denser element; more *yin*; moistens and nourishes brain, bone marrow, and lubricates joints. Sweat, snivel, tears, drool, and spittle.
Both elements are also partly responsible for blood quality and quantity.

Dysfunction

Damage to Body Fluids

Body fluids are *yin* and deficiencies always appear as dryness (advanced stage = exsiccosis).

Symptoms
Dry skin, lips, nose, tongue, mucous membranes, or mouth; dry cough; constipation.

Nutritional Therapy
Moisten dryness with pear, apple, tangerine, soy milk, tofu, milk, wheat, tomato, coconut milk, grapes, peanuts, and pine nuts.

Body Fluid Accumulation

Dampness caused by a deficiency of spleen *qi*, lung *qi*, or kidney *qi*, or of all three organs.

Nutritional Therapy

Primarily supplement spleen network with millet, rice, fennel, potatoes, and honey.

Organ	Symptom
Lung	Edemas in upper part of body, face, hands
Spleen	Edemas in center part of body, abdomen, ascites
Kidney	Edemas in lower part of body, legs, ankles

Nutritional Therapy

Disperse dampness with amaranth, barley, corn silk tea, ginger, dandelion, and soy milk.

Causes of Diseases

TCM views health as a dynamic balance between *yin* and *yang*. Disease develops when this balance is disturbed. TCM generally distinguishes between "external" and "internal" pathogenic factors that can cause disharmony of *yin* and *yang*.

Other causes of diseases are:

- **Constitution:** Quality of inherited congenital constitution (*jing*), constitution of mother during pregnancy, birth events and miscarriages.
- **Diet:** Malnutrition or excess, inferior-quality diet, imbalanced diet, poor eating habits.
- **Unbalanced lifestyle:** Overwork, stress, physical, mental, or emotional strain, lack of exercise, sexual problems.
- Trauma
- Parasites
- Treatment errors

External Bioclimatic Factors or Impediments

Depending on the source used, the impediments (synonym: *bi lun*, or adverse climates) include:

- Wind impediment
- Cold impediment
- Damp impediment
- Heat impediment
- Dryness

These impediments often coincide and attack the body by entering the channels and causing "external illnesses." For example, wind-cold can cause the flu.

In many climates of the Northern hemisphere, wind-cold and damp are among the most common external pathogenic factors. When applied early, nutritional therapy provides excellent opportunities for compensating attacks by external bioclimatic factors.

Wind

Disorders caused by wind (draft) have *yang* energy and appear suddenly, often serving as a kind of "carrier" to transport cold or heat to the outer layer of the body. This injures the outer layers, especially the *yang* channels of the upper half of the body.

Symptoms

Sneezing, shivering, colds, running nose, fever, joint pain, headache, aversion to wind and cold, sudden change of symptoms.

Nutritional Therapy

Expulsion of wind or wind-cold.

For wind-cold: Acrid spices, especially ginger, green onions, garlic, coriander.

For wind-heat: Celery stalk, eggplant, water chestnut, green tea, watermelon.

Cold

Cold, another important pathogenic factor with *yin* quality, is divided into external and internal cold.

External cold, caused by external exposure to cold (winter, air conditioning), results in *qi* and blood stagnation, and manifests itself, for example, in fixed, cold-dependent pain.

Internal cold, caused by the excessive consumption of cold foods or a deep penetration of external cold, results in *qi* and blood stagnation and a weakening of the zang organs.

Symptoms

Freezing, cold extremities, and, in case of deeply penetrating cold, joint pain, arthritis, gastrointestinal disorders, diarrhea, vomiting, and abdominal pain that improves with warmth.

Nutritional Therapy

Dispersion of cold with acrid spices such as ginger, green onions, garlic, coriander, chili, black pepper, fennel, chicken, lamb, alcohol.

Dampness

Dampness is an external pathogenic factor that stems from damp weather conditions, wet surroundings, or wet clothing. Internally, dampness forms as a result of spleen/pancreas network dysfunction. When it becomes chronic, it presents as mucous membrane symptoms.
Damp diseases have a pronounced *yin* character, with qualities such as heaviness, stickiness, swelling, slowing of normal *qi* flow, and a tendency toward long-term illness.

Symptoms

Chronic fatigue, feeling of heaviness in head and limbs, dizziness, edemas, dyspnea (shortness of breath), tightness in chest, and abdominal symptoms such as loss of appetite, nausea, vomiting, diarrhea.
Damp weather is often associated with a worsening of symptoms.

Nutritional Therapy

Dispelling and drying up dampness.
Dampness/heat: Mung beans, soy milk, dandelion, corn silk tea, seaweed.
Dampness: Barley, millet, ginger, carp, green tea.

Heat

Heat is a pathogenic factor with *yang* character. Because heat has a tendency to rise, it primarily interferes with the upper parts of the body. Heat dries out and harms *yin*. It also harms blood and body fluids and impacts the spirit (*shen*).

Symptoms

Restlessness, irritability, nervousness, sleep disorders, insomnia, hyperactivity, delirium, itching, red rashes, fever, thirst, dry mouth and lips, reddened, sore throat.

Nutritional Therapy

Clear heat and cool, moisten; replenish body fluids with tomatoes, dandelion, cucumbers, watermelon, wheat, tofu, mung beans, sprouts, orange, lemon, banana, kiwi fruit, crayfish, rabbit, salt, green tea, and yogurt.

Dryness (*Zao*)

Dryness is a *yang* factor and often appears in combination with heat. Heat, however, plays a more significant role. Dryness damages the lung and harms *yin* and body fluids.

Symptoms

Dry, scaly skin; chapped lips, dry cough, little saliva, thirst, constipation and exsiccosis.

Nutritional Therapy

Moisten and replenish body fluids with pear, banana, watermelon, tangerine, soy milk, tofu, wheat, peanut, honey, cow's milk, butter, and yogurt.

Internal Factors, "The Five Minds (Emotions)" (*Wu Shi*)

The five minds are **joy**, **anger**, **anxiety**, **thought**, and **fear**. Excess or lack of emotions damages health by producing specific reactions in the bowels and viscera (*zang fu*) of the body. Protracted emotional imbalance can lead to serious and deep organ dysfunctions. Dietary measures can help by cooling or warming the corresponding networks of emotions (e.g., sadness/thought—lung network).

- Sadness (sad thoughts) and anxiety harms the lungs
- Fear harms the kidneys
- Anger and rage harm the liver
- Excessive joy or stress harm the heart
- Worry, brooding, and excessive thought (mental activity) harm the spleen

Traditional Chinese Nutrition Theory

The beginnings of Chinese dietetics can be traced back to the *Zhou* Dynasty (1100–700 BC). At the time, four groups of healers were responsible for providing medical care:

- Therapists for nutritional matters (dieticians): *shi yi*
- Therapists for internal diseases (internists): *ji yi*
- Therapists for external illnesses and injuries (surgeons): *yang yi*
- Therapists for sick animals (veterinarians): *shou yi*

Dieticians were the most significant of these healers. Their task was primarily the prevention of disease in their patients, along with therapeutic use of diet for acute and chronic diseases.

The root of the term "diet" reveals an interesting connection between the original Western perception of the term and the Asian concept.

Diet is derived from the Greek term "diaita," meaning life care, lifestyle, or way of life. Lifestyle highlights an aspect that resembles "Tao," the connection of humans and nature.

With its emphasis on prevention, dietary therapy in TCM enabled dieticians to be solely responsible for the health care of entire families of dignitaries. Health was achieved through diet.

Prevention, the avoidance of diseases, plays an important role in all TCM therapies. The value placed on prevention is illustrated by an ancient Chinese system of wages for physicians (this may be an anecdote!).

The amount of a physician's annual salary was determined by the immaculate state of health displayed by their patients. The less their patients fell sick, the higher their salary.

Acupuncture, moxibustion, phytotherapy, dietetics, and exercise (*qi gong, tai chi*) are the foundations of therapy in TCM.

Even in its origins, dietetics was assigned a vital role in the treatment of disease. To quote from the *Su Wen*:

> *"When the body is too weak, the therapist should use foods to replenish the deficit."*

The famous physician *Sun Si Miao* of the *Tang* Dynasty (AD 618–907) further emphasized the important role of dietary therapy:

> *"Dietary therapy should be the first step when one treats a disease. Only when this is unsuccessful should one try medicines."*

In a further quote, he emphasizes the preventive character of Chinese dietetics:

> *"Without the knowledge of proper diet, it is hardly possible to enjoy good health."*

Nutritional therapy offers the following options:

- "Life care"—Tao
- Prevention of disease
- Therapy for acute disease
- Therapy for chronic disease

The *Qi* Energy Concept of TCM

Qi, the life force, or life energy, is of primary importance in TCM.

Sufficient and freely coursing *qi* signifies vitality, health, and the body's capacities. *Qi* vacuity lowers overall quality of life and encourages development of disease.

The body gathers its daily energy from three sources.

The Three Energy Sources

- Congenital constitution essence (*jing*)
- *Gu qi* (drum *qi*) from food
- Ancestral (air) *qi* (*zong qi*)

Congenital Constitution Essence (*Jing*)

The inherited essence of the parents, stored in the kidneys, provides the basis for all life processes and maturation processes in the body. Quantity and quality of *jing* are determined at birth. Since this energy reserve can not be replenished, Chi-

nese physicians recommend careful management of this potential. As little *jing* as possible should be used to meet one's daily energy requirement.
Note: Dissipated, excessive lifestyles, an overactive sex life, hard drugs, extreme stress or strain, and fasting diminish and weaken *jing*.

Gu Qi (Drum *Qi*, or Food *Qi*)

Gu qi develops during the first transformation stage as stomach and spleen process ingested foods. The quality of newly formed *gu qi* depends on the purity of foods ingested (if possible, fresh and not processed or denatured) and on the condition of the digestive organs stomach and spleen. If these organs are in a chronic or acute state of fatigue, quantity and quality of *gu qi* are reduced. This gradually leads to general debility with a tendency to chronic vacuity symptoms.
Since *gu qi* is a renewable energy source, it plays a key role in Chinese medicine. *Gu qi* makes up the biggest share of the renewable energies. This role was emphasized by the traditional "School of the Middle," which viewed nutritional therapy as a key element in the treatment of diseases.

"Without knowledge about proper diet, it is hardly possible to enjoy good health."

Ancestral (Air) *Qi* (*Zong Qi*)

With each breath, ancestral *qi* contributes to the total energy of the body, making up about one third of the total renewable energy. Proper breathing and good, clean air enhance its energetic quality. Ancient Chinese techniques can contribute to an increase in ancestral *qi* through specific breathing exercises, such as *qi gong* or *tai chi*, or exercises from the Asian martial arts.

The three energy sources congenital essence (jing), gu qi (drum qi), and ancestral qi (zong qi) merge into true qi (zhen qi), which flows through the body in channels as construction qi (ying qi) and defense qi (wei qi).

These basic concepts highlight the need for TCM therapy to encompass several complementary therapeutic principles.
Acupuncture especially influences true *qi* (*zhen qi*). However, acupuncture, with the exception of moxibustion, does not supplement *qi* in a patient: instead it moves *qi*, balances it, and disperses stagnation.

Tip: Before employing acupuncture treatment for *qi*, *yang*, or *yin* vacuity, please note that *qi* vacuity or *yang* vacuity require expanded treatment modalities involving dietary measures and Chinese herbs to supplement *qi*, *yang*, body fluids, and blood. Successful treatment of *yin* vacuity requires replenishing the physical body and its substance with dietary and herbal therapy. These build the foundation for effective acupuncture treatment.

The Concept of *Qi* Production

Prenatal essence (*jing*)
about 5 %

Food essence (*gu qi*)
about 70 %

Air essence (*zong qi*)
about 25 %

True *qi* (*zeng qi*)

Channel *qi* (*ying qi*)

Defense *qi* (*wei qi*)

Possible Therapeutic Approaches

Prenatal essence (*jing*)
about 1–5 %
(virtually nonrenewable,
hence protect: lifestyle, diet)

Food essence (*gu qi*)
about 70 %
(primarily diet, accompanied
by phytotherapy and
acupuncture)

Air essence (*zong qi*)
about 25 %
(*qi gong*, *tai chi*)

True *qi* (*zheng qi*)
(diet, phytotherapy, *qi gong*)

Channel *qi* (*ying qi*)
(acupuncture and moxibustion)

Defense *qi* (*wei qi*)
(acupuncture and moxibustion)

Function of the Triple Burner (*San Jiao*)

In TCM, the triple burner (*san jiao*) is likened to the "official responsible for irrigation and control of waterways" in a feudal state.

The *Nei Jing* describes the triple burner's main task as the creation, transformation, and movement of body fluids (*jin ye*), with an emphasis on digestion and excretion.

The triple burner coordinates distribution and movement of the different types of *qi* to ensure continuous support of organ networks and enable unobstructed movement of *qi*. Disorders appear as accumulation of fluids, such as edemas and urinary retention.

In Western perception, the triple burner reflects the anatomical division of the body into three parts, described in historic texts such as the *Nan Jing* (The Classic of Difficult Issues) and the *Ling Shu* (second part of the *Huang Di Nei Jing:* The Yellow Emperor's Classic of Medicine).

The Upper Burner:
Heart, lungs, pericardium,
upward from diaphragm

The lungs unite ancestral *qi* (*zong qi*) with *gu qi* (drum *qi*) to form true *qi* (*zhen qi*), which flows in the channels, and distribute true *qi* through the body. Lungs and heart use *qi* to "breathe life" into the blood (*xue*) of the upper burner.

The lungs disperse fluids as a "fine mist" that moistens skin and muscles. The upper burner controls upward movement and defense *qi*.

The Center Burner:
Spleen, pancreas, stomach,
between diaphragm and navel

In classic texts, the center burner is often compared to a boiling kettle, or a fermentation barrel that absorbs food as "foam" and processes it. Stomach and spleen are responsible for proper transformation and transport of food. This process separates "clear" (*qing*) from "turbid" (*zhuo*). The spleen moves clear *qi* into the upper burner. Turbid *qi* is sent downward through the stomach. Once food has been transformed, the flow of essential *qi* (*jing qi*) derived from clear food is directed upward, toward lung and heart.

This system provides the body with the main share of renewable *qi* as well as with blood (*xue*) and body fluids (*jin ye*), which are moved along from there. The center burner is central to Chinese nutrition: An appropriate and sufficient diet strengthens spleen *qi* daily and protects the energy resources of the kidney network.

The quality of food provided to the center burner determines the body's entire energy store, as well as quality and quantity of blood and body fluids.

The Lower Burner:
Liver, kidney, bladder, and intestine,
downward from navel

The lower burner is usually described as a "swamp" or "sewer." Its main function is the transformation and excretion of fluids and waste products. The flow of *qi* is directed downward.

B Methodology of Nutritional Therapy

Energetics of Food

Western nutrition theory focuses on the analytical and quantitative categorization of foods. This categorization is based on material food components such as carbohydrates, fat, protein, vitamins, minerals, and trace elements.

The Eastern view, on the other hand, follows the qualitative, holistic concept of *yin* and *yang* and illustrates how thermal nature and flavor of foods and medicinal herbs influence the body.

Hippocrates and Hildegard von Bingen employed similar qualitative, more energetically oriented approaches. They used diet as an important and inexpensive source of therapy for sustaining health and treating disease.

TCM makes a close connection between foods and medicinal herbs for therapy, since their classification follows the same criteria. Foods and herbs can both promote and impede each other in their effect on the body. For example, it would be pointless to prescribe phlegm-reducing herbs and acupuncture to patients without informing them about phlegm-producing foods such as fatty foods, "junk food," excess dairy products, alcohol, etc. Effective "holistic" therapy in such cases needs to include dietary measures, for example phlegm-reducing foods such as pears.

Four basic criteria for energetic classification of foods

- **Thermal nature:** Hot, warm, neutral, cool, cold
- **Flavor:** Sweet, acrid, sour, bitter, salty
- **Organ network:** Spleen, stomach, lung, large intestine, kidney, bladder, liver, gallbladder, heart, small intestine
- **Direction of movement:** Upbearing, floating, downbearing, falling

In the classic "Recipes Worth a Thousand Pieces of Gold" (quian jin fang), the famous Chinese physician Sun Si Miao states: "For the body to retain its balance and harmony requires only following a proper diet. One should never take medications in an uncontrolled manner. The power of medications is one-sided, and there are cases in which they are helpful."

Energetic classification assigns foods primarily to four areas: thermal nature, flavor, organ network, and direction of movement. These are modeled after paradigms rooted in the empirical foundations of TCM.

Tip: **Thermal nature and flavor are of principal value in Chinese nutritional therapy. Flavor and thermal nature are often combined to describe a flavor and its effect on the body, e.g., sweet–hot or sour–cool.**

General preventive nutrition can focus on only the thermal nature or flavor of foods. Nutritional therapy designed to heal illness, however, needs to be based on a firm diagnosis by a TCM practitioner and consider all four criteria (thermal nature, flavor, organ network, and direction).

Energetic Thermal Nature

Foods are divided into five energetic temperature levels:

Hot, warm = *yang*
Cold, cool = *yin*
Neutral

Foods and their Thermal Nature

Food category	Hot	Warm	Neutral	Cold	Cool
Beverages	Alcohol (high –proof) Yogi tea	Cocoa Coffee Red wine		Water	Black tea Fruit juices Peppermint tea Sour milk Soy milk Wheat beer
Condiments and sweeteners			Honey	Salt Soy sauce	
Dairy products		Butter Goat's cheese	Cow's milk cheese		Yogurt
Eggs, fish, fowl, meat, etc.	Lamb	Beef Chicken Eel Salmon	Carp Duck Chicken egg Goose Pork	Shrimp Crayfish	Rabbit
Fruit and vegetables		Cherry Fennel Leek Peach Onion	Carrot Cauliflower Grape Fig Plum Potato	Asparagus Banana Orange Rhubarb Seaweed Tomato Watermelon	Celery Cucumber Soy bean Sprouts Spinach Zucchini
Grains and legumes			Corn Lentil Millet Peas Rice Spelt		Barley Tofu Wheat
Herbs and spices	Cinnamon Chili Curry Garlic Ginger Paprika Pepper	Anise Basil Rosemary		Dandelion Yellow gentian	Tarragon
Seeds and nuts		Walnut	Hazelnut		

This same classification is applied to Chinese medicinal herbs and is rooted in a 3000-year tradition of Chinese medicine based on application, observation, experience, and intuition.
Independent of its preparation, every food has a "natural" energetic, basic thermal nature that has a specific effect on the body.

Example
Energetically "hot" foods such as pepper, chili, and garlic have a heating, warming effect on the body. "Cold" foods such as tomatoes and bananas cool the body. Warm and cool foods have a milder effect on the body. Neutral foods do not change the energetic level of the body.
Thermal quality initially has a general effect on the body: it cools or warms it. Flavor and association with one of the five phases determine the food's effect on a particular organ or network.

Example
The sweet flavor is associated with the earth phase and primarily influences the corresponding organs stomach and spleen. It has a warming or cooling effect on stomach/spleen, depending on thermal nature: Fennel tea warms the stomach, while bananas have a cooling effect.

Hot

Hot foods increase *yang*, speed up *qi*, activate, warm, disperse, move upward and outward, warm the bowels and viscera (*zang fu*), eliminate external and internal cold, and mobilize defense energy.

Example
"Treatment of cold symptoms":
➢ Ginger, cinnamon, lamb, chili

! Excess creates heat (*yang* repletion), injures *yin*, and dries out body fluids.

Warm

Warm foods strengthen *yang* and *qi*, warm the body, bowels and viscera (*zang fu*), and warm and strengthen the center burner.

Example
"Treatment of cold symptoms":
➢ Fennel, chicken, beef, oats

! Excess creates *yang* repletion.

Neutral

Neutral foods build up *qi* and body fluids, and stabilize and harmonize the body.

Example
"Treatment of *qi* vacuity":
➢ Honey, rice, potatoes

Cool

Cool foods supplement body fluids (*jin ye*) and blood (*xue*), slow down *qi*, and clear heat.

Example
"Treatment of heat symptoms":
➢ Yogurt, soy milk, wheat

Cold

Cold foods create cold, cool internal heat, and have a calming effect on the spirit (*shen*).

Example
"Treatment of heat symptoms":
➢ Watermelon, dandelion, orange

! Excess damages *qi* and *yang*, and thoroughly cools down the body.

Therapeutic goals are derived from the *yin–yang* principle. The *Nei Jing* states.

"If something is cold, heat it. If something is hot, cool it." Supplementing the opposite polarity restores original balance.

Cold requires warmth
= yang (hot and warm)
Heat requires cold
= yin (cold and cool)

"*Yang* Foods"

"*Yang* foods" are hot or warm foods; they warm and invigorate the body.

Acrid spices (pepper, garlic, cinnamon)
Meat (beef, chicken, game/venison, lamb)
Coffee
Alcohol
Oats
Cherry, peach

Yang foods are recommended for disorders of a cool or cold nature, for example:

Qi Vacuity

Symptoms
Fatigue, pale complexion, shivering, loss of appetite, susceptibility to infection.

Yang Vacuity

Symptoms
Cold dominates, chronic cold hands and feet, exhaustion, lethargy, sloppy stool, frequent urge to urinate with pale urine.

"*Yin* Foods"

Yin foods are cool or cold foods; they have a cooling, soothing effect on the body.

Dairy products
Fruit (especially tropical fruit like banana, citrus fruit)
Mineral water
Tomato
Wheat

Yin foods are important therapy for heat disorders, for example:

Yin Vacuity

Symptoms
Dry mucous membranes, dry tongue, night sweat, hot hands and feet, feeling hot in the afternoon.

Yang Repletion

Symptoms
Loud voice, red face, restlessness, hectic, hyperactive, sleep disorders, feeling hot.

Example

Practical Application

Patient is lethargic, pale, tired, shivering.

Diagnosis: *Yang* vacuity
Therapy: Replenish *yang* with *yang* foods (energetically hot or warm foods like lamb, beef, pepper, fennel tea).

Patient is agitated, irritable, with red complexion and sudden headaches.

Diagnosis: *Yang* repletion.
Therapy: Drain *yang* repletion, clear heat with *yin* foods (energetically cool or cold foods like fruits, salad, peppermint tea, tomato).

The Five Flavors (*Wu Wei*)

Sweet—acrid—salty—sour—bitter

Organization of Flavors into *Yin*, *Yang*, and Organ Network		
Yang quality	**Phase**	**Network**
Sweet	Earth	Spleen /stomach
Acrid	Metal	Lung/large intestine
Yin quality	**Phase**	**Network**
Bitter	Fire	Heart /small intestine
Salty	Water	Kidney/bladder
Sour	Wood	Liver /gallbladder

Food Classification According to Flavor

Sweet	Acrid	Salty	Sour	Bitter
Almond	Celeriac (celery root)	Crayfish	Adzuki beans	Basil
Apple	Chili	Duck	Apple	Chicory
Anise	Cinnamon	Ham	Apricot	Celeriac (celery root)
Barley	Fennel	Oyster	Grape	Coffee
Banana	Garlic	Octopus	Kiwi	Dandelion
Beef	Ginger	Pork	Lemon	Lettuce
Butter	Kohlrabi	Pigeon	Mango	Parsley
Carrot	Onion	Salt	Orange	Tea
Cheese	Paprika	Soy sauce	Plum	Tobacco
Chicken	Pepper		Pineapple	
Corn	Radishes		Cheese	
Duck	Thyme		Curd cheese	
Eggplant Fennel	Watercress		Farmer's cheese	
Fig			Cream cheese	
Milk			Sour (curdled) milk	
Millet			Tomato	
Oats				
Pork				
Potato				
Pumpkin				
Pear				
Rabbit				
Rice				
Spinach				
Wheat				

The five flavors are the oldest system of food classification in TCM and are mentioned in the *Nei Jing*. Flavors can be divided according to their *yin* or *yang* quality.

***Yang* quality: Sweet, acrid**
***Yin* quality: Salty, sour, bitter**

In addition to their specific *yin*/*yang* effect, the five flavors each belong to one of the five phases. Thus each flavor is closely associated with the organ network linked to the phase influenced by the flavor.

Phase	Network
Sweet	Spleen/stomach
Acrid	Lung/large intestine
Salty	Kidney/bladder
Sour	Liver/gallbladder
Bitter	Heart/small intestine

Each flavor also has other important qualities that influence the body:

Sweet Flavor

Phase
Earth

Network
Spleen/stomach

Effect
Warming, strengthening, harmonizing, relaxing, and moistening. Sweet has the strongest supplementing effect on the body (craving for "sweets" following heavy physical, emotional, or mental exertion).

General Application
Sweet flavor strengthens primarily spleen *qi*, where it builds up energy. It also helps with acute weakness (ravishing appetite). With its moistening effect, sweet foods nourish body fluids, relieve inner tension (compulsive eating, overeating due to emotional stress), and stabilize one's "inner center" (earth phase).

! Excess sweet flavors harm spleen *qi* and produce pathogenic dampness. This can, over time, lead to phlegm disorders, for example recurrent bronchitis, sinusitis, chronic fatigue, dull sensation in head. The *Nei Jing* says: *"Sweet flavor adds flesh,"* resulting in obesity and weakness of connective tissue. Via the controlling cycles, excess sweet flavor can weaken the kidneys, resulting in bone and teeth disorders.

Acrid Flavor

Phase
Metal

Network
Lung/large intestine

Effect
Moves *qi*, invigorates energy circulation, loosens stagnation, disperses, opens pores, frees surface of exogenous disease factors, and produces perspiration.

General Application
The acrid flavor strengthens the lungs and banishes exogenous disease factors, especially wind–cold. Its sweat-producing effect and ability to open pores are helpful during the acute stage of a cold (ginger). Moderately spicy foods during the winter months offer excellent protection against colds. Due to their invigorating effect on *qi*, acrid flavors loosen emotional stagnation and associated breathing problems (tightness in chest). With its tendency to move *qi* upward, acrid flavors are beneficial when experiencing emotional strain, such as sadness, melancholy, and despondency (emotions of the lung network).

! **People with heat symptoms should assiduously avoid acrid flavors!** Excess causes heat symptoms and can impair the skin (dryness, allergies, itching skin, sun allergy). Through the controlling cycles, acrid flavors can damage mostly liver and gallbladder (ascendant liver *yang*, or *gan yang shang kang*, for example irritability, hyperactivity, sleep disorders.) Acrid flavors disperse spirit (*shen*), resulting in inner restlessness, hyperactivity, and sleep disorders. Via the engendering (*sheng*) cycle, kidney essence may overheat, causing exaggerated sexual desire, sexual compulsions. May weaken muscle tone and cause dryness in large intestine (constipation).

Salty Flavor

Phase
Water

Network
Kidney/bladder

Effect
Cools, moistens, downbears, softens, loosens

General Application
Salty flavor in moderation supplements kidney function, promotes urine and stool excretion (Epsom salt), dissolves congestions and hardened areas (e.g., subcutaneous nodules, phlegm accumulation).

More salt restriction, excess is common! Dehydrates body; damages fluids, blood, and vascular system (hypertension); hardens muscles and damages bones. Via the restraining cycle (*ke*), inhibits heart and spirit (*shen*), decreases mental abilities, and leads to rigid thinking.

Sour Flavor

Phase
Wood

Network
Liver/gallbladder

Effect
Astringent, gathers and preserves fluids

General Application
Sour-cooling foods refresh the body, reduce excessive perspiration, promote the creation of fluids, and soothe "heated" temperaments by cooling emotional "heat" in the liver/gallbladder.
Sour flavor also supplements *yin*. "Sour makes happy." In times of emotional stress and anger, the sour flavor should be favored, because it supplements liver *yin*. The supplementing effect of sour flavors is moved along to the heart element (via the engendering *sheng* cycle).
Sour moves inward and is healing for distracted, unfocused minds or restless lifestyles.

Sour flavor is contraindicated when acute external weather conditions (wind-cold) impact the body. When pathogenic effects are still located in the outer layers of the body, sour flavors pull these factors into deeper layers. This worsens the course of disease and reduces treatment success (no heated lemon juice during acute cold!). The therapy of choice for colds is acrid flavors, which open pores, promote perspiration, and clear pathogenic factors from the body surface.

Excess sour flavors damage muscle tone (lowering pH > sore muscles, muscle contraction) and sinews and should be avoided when suffering from nonarticular rheumatism and arthritis.

Bitter Flavor

Phase
Fire

Network
Heart/small intestine

Effect
Drying, hardening, downbearing

General Application
Bitter-cool, downbears and supports the body's digestive and excretion functions (digestive teas with amaroids/bitters, such as gallbladder tea, wormwood tea). It supplements heart *yin* and has a calming effect, especially following stress and mental strain (beer, especially light-colored wheat beer). Bitter-warm flavors in the form of aperitifs, or bitter liqueurs, stimulate the digestive organs due to their alcohol content, especially in combination with bitter flavors.
Engendering (*sheng*) cycle: Bitter (fire) supplements spleen/pancreas and stomach (earth). Its drying property prevents the formation of damp throughout the body. When taken in appropriate dosages, bitter is a spleen *qi* tonic, preferably during moist-cool weather (coffee, red wine).

Too much bitter–cool has a strong laxative effect and causes diarrhea (Epsom salt). Excess bitter–warm flavors (coffee!) dehydrate (dry skin), damage fluids (especially blood vacuity, poor circulation), damage texture (*Nei Jing*: *"Bitter spreads to the bones"*), heat up the heart, and inhibit spirit. In Western medicine, coffee is considered a "calcium robber" and promotes osteoporosis.

Via the engendering (*sheng*) cycle, surplus heat in the fire phase is moved into the earth phase, where it can cause damage to spleen/stomach.
A symptom often seen in practice is "stomach heat" (TCM), in Western medicine known as gastritis or ulcer, caused by excessive coffee consumption, nicotine, or stress (TCM: stress = heat).

Tip: **Green tea is energetically "cool," while black tea is more neutral in thermal nature.**

Flavor Association with Organ Networks

Along with their general effect, each of the five flavors is associated with one of the five phases. This explains the flavor's effect on the specific bowels and viscera (*zang fu*) of a corresponding phase. The *Nei Jing* states:

"Sourness enters the liver, bitterness enters the heart, sweetness enters the spleen, acridity enters the lungs, saltiness enters the kidneys." It goes on to say: "Sourness enters the sinews, bitterness enters the blood, acridity enters qi, sweetness enters the flesh, saltiness enters the bones." (Huang Di Nei Ling Shui Zu Yi: The Yellow Emperor's Classic of Medicine)

Phase	Flavor	Organ
Earth	Sweet	Spleen/stomach
Metal	Acrid	Lung/large instestine
Water	Salty	Kidney/bladder
Wood	Sour	Liver/gallbladder
Fire	Bitter	Heart/small instestine

Food Table: Organ Networks

Viscera (zang organs)	**Spleen**	**Lungs**	**Kidney**	**Liver**	**Heart**
	Anise Beef Caraway seed Carrots Chicken Fig Honey Millet Oats Pork Rice Salmon	Almond Duck Garlic Radish Pepper Peppermint tea Watercress	Chestnut Grape Lamb Millet Oats Oyster Plum Raspberry Venison Wheat Walnuts	Alcohol Celery stalks Eel Liver Garlic Lemon Peppermint tea Rye Wheat	Alcohol Black tea Chili Coffee Dandelion Gentian Wheat
Bowels (fu organs)	**Stomach**	**Large intestine**	**Bladder**	**Gallbladder**	**Small intestine**
	Beef Caraway seed Carrots Chamomile tea Chicken Corn Fennel Fig Honey Millet Pork Rice Trout	Banana Corn Pepper Rabbit Spinach Tofu Wheat germ	Caraway seed Fennel Parsley Squid	Belgian endive Mung bean Peach Rye	Green lettuce Mushroom Snail Spinach

Note: In each network, some food flavors can influence bowels and viscera (*zang fu*) in five thermal directions.

Example

Sweet–cold, banana: Clears stomach heat
Sweet–warm, carrot: Warms stomach
Sweet–hot, anise schnapps: Warms, heats stomach

Example: Carrot

Flavor
Sweet

Phase
Earth

Thermal Nature
Warm

Network
Stomach and spleen/stomach

Effect
Warms and strengthens primarily the digestive organs stomach and spleen/pancreas. Useful for loss of appetite, nausea, digestive stagnation, constipation, and diarrhea.

Qi Movement Caused by Food: Food Direction

This quality describes how a food influences the movement of *qi* in the body.

Upbearing Movement

Foods that move *yang* upward mainly have sweet–acrid flavors and moderate thermal nature (warm, neutral); recommended for use during spring season.

Example
Green onion, garlic, alcoholic beverages

Floating Movement

Moves *qi* upward and outward (sweating), expels external pathogenic factors, dissipates cold and wind; strong (warm/hot) thermal nature, sweet and acrid flavor.

Example
Cinnamon, pepper, high-proof alcoholic beverages

Downbearing Movement

Moves *qi* downward and inward, retains *qi* and body fluids on the inside; cooling–neutral thermal nature, primarily sour flavor, partly bitter and salty. For example, downbearing ascending liver *yang* with dizziness, headaches.

Example
Yogurt, lemon

Falling Movement

Moves downward, has a laxative or diuretic effect, and a cooling, mostly cold thermal nature, with strong salty or bitter flavor.

Example
Crayfish, Epsom salt

Influencing the Thermal Nature of Foods

Chinese dietetics recognizes over 50 different ways of preparing foods. The ways in which foods are heated or prepared exert the most significant influence on the *qi* or thermal nature of foods. Preparation methods can be divided into two categories.

Cooling Cooking Methods

These methods increase the cooling nature of foods. They can cool down warm or hot foods by using refreshing or cold ingredients. Cooling cooking methods increase the *yin* potential of meals.

Cooling cooking methods include:
Blanching, steaming, salting (pickling in brine), boiling in plentiful water, and preparation using refreshing ingredients such as fruit, tropical fruit, or sprouts.

Warming Cooking Methods

These methods support the warming effect of foods and reduce the refreshing (cooling) effect of foods. Warming cooking methods increase the *yang* potential of meals.

Warming cooking methods include:
Grilling, frying, roasting, smoking, searing, baking, long simmering in liquid, cooking with alcohol, using hot or warming spices.

Cooking Methods in Detail

Baking △△▽

This cooking method gently supplies *yang* energy to foods. It is useful for avoiding the cooling effect of refreshing or strongly cooling foods (*yin* foods, e.g., vegetables). Baking foods or making casseroles is a way for vegetarians to supply their body with *yang* energy and balance the cooling effect of the *yin* foods that make up the biggest share of a vegetarian diet. Baking is beneficial for supplying the body with *yang* energy during the cold season. Vegetables or raw foods, which due to their *yin* character cool the body, can become warming through baking. For example, baked tomatoes or baked apples.

Blanching △▽

This method of preparation does not change the energy level of a food, but foods become easier to digest when heated.

Frying and Roasting △△▽

Frying and roasting supply foods with *yang* energy. A good variation of this method in Chinese cooking is the use of a wok with little or no oil added. "Woking" brings foods in contact with extreme heat for a short time only and lends them an outer crunchy layer, but leaves them juicy and fresh on the inside. This provides foods with strong *yang* energy on the outside and a balancing *yin* component on the inside.

Frying and roasting should be avoided with internal heat symptoms. Using too much oil or other frying fats can also develop moist heat, which strains the liver/gallbladder organ network.

Steaming △▽

Steaming changes the thermal nature of foods very little, which classifies this method as neutral.

Grilling/Broiling/Barbecue △△△△

Grilling, broiling, or barbecuing develops a strong *yang* effect. Direct contact with a heat source supplies foods with intense heat. This develops a strong warming effect in grilled foods, especially meat. Because grilling, broiling, or barbecuing may develop toxic substances in foods, this method should be applied only in exceptional cases.

Grilling broiling, or barbecuing should be avoided with heat symptoms.

Boiling/Simmering △▽ → △△▽

With boiling, the warming effect is determined by cooking time and temperature. Brief boiling adds little *yang* energy to foods. Prolonged boiling over several hours (up to 36 hours for the Master Soup) develops immense *yang* potential in foods. In TCM, this heightened energy potential is much more important than any potential loss of vitamins during prolonged cooking. Stews containing warming meats and simmered for long periods are an excellent foundation for restoring *yang* potential in a person with *qi* or *yin* vacuity. Boiling is also valuable during cold winter months (meat, broths, and vegetable soups). This cooking method is no longer common in many parts of the world, but it is very effective for healing in Chinese medicine. In the past, boiling or simmering for long periods was widespread in Europe, especially in Northern Europe, where, for days on end, a pot would simmer over an open fire, with new food items added regularly. These energetically very warm meals provided the necessary balance for frequently cool weather conditions.

Tip: "The Master Soup" △△△▽▽

In Chinese nutrition, the energetics of a food are influenced by cooking duration and intensity of supplied heat. So-called Master Soups, which simmer over a low heat for between six and 36 hours, are of special significance here. These soups are believed by traditional practitioners of TCM to contain tremendous healing powers. In TCM, the Master Soup is used to treat general *qi* vacuity or *yang* vacuity, and is recommended particularly after long, strenuous illnesses, during recovery, as well as following childbirth to boost strength in the new mother. Prolonged cooking increases the warming and strengthening effect of meat and bones. Vegetarian stews experience more of an energetic devaluation as a result of extended cooking times. Warming spices should be used instead of prolonged cooking for vegetarian stews to increase the energetics of the meal.

Example
Selection of specific ingredients can determine the effect on the organ network:

- Lentil stew with pork supplements the kidney network.
- Carrot stew with beef supplements the stomach/spleen network.

Cooking with Alcohol △△

Alcohol not only enhances the flavor of foods, it also warms them. The movement pattern of alcohol is upbearing, which pulls *yang* upward. Alcohol also dissolves stagnation, promotes *qi* and blood circulation, and dissipates cold. This can balance *qi* vacuity in the upper burner. Cooking with alcohol warms the center burner (stomach and spleen) and the upper burner (heart and lung). During emotional strains with downbearing *qi*, such as dejection, resignation, or sadness, meals cooked with alcohol upbear *qi* and enhance mood. Cooking with alcohol warms meals, increases the body's energy, and stimulates *qi* circulation in the body, which can also loosen emotional blockage and tension.

Boiling with Plentiful Water ▽▽

This method reduces the *yang* energy of foods, especially in vegetables, and is not recommend.

Cooking with Cooling Ingredients ▽ (e.g., Fruit, Sprouts)

Using cooling ingredients during cooking balances excessive *yang* parts (such as meat) and harmonizes the meal as a whole.

Slow, Gentle Frying (Braising) △

Braising with high-quality vegetable oil supplies only a moderate amount of heat.

Salting (Pickling in Brine) ▽

Salt lowers food *qi* and has a cold thermal nature. By reducing the *yang* energy of foods, salting increases *yin* energy.

Smoking △△

Smoking supplies foods with *yang* energy, but less than with grilling. Smoked fish is recommended as a kidney supplement during colder months. Smoked foods should be used rather sparingly, especially in conjunction with excess salt.

Seasoning △△

The thermal nature of most spices is either hot or warm. Spices not only season foods, but also have a strong energetic effect on them. They supplement and warm stomach and spleen. From a Chinese medicine point of view, this explains the digestion-promoting effect of many spices. By using warming spices such as bay leaf, caraway, or cloves, many *yin* vegetables like red cabbage, white cabbage, or sauerkraut become easier to digest. Long cooking also contributes to this effect. Highly seasoned foods strongly influence the body's energy level and should be reduced or avoided during repletion states or inner heat. For example, energetically hot coffee can be unfavorable with sleep disorders, which are a symptom of internal heat. Sleep disturbances can be provoked by the consumption of acrid spices like garlic, onion, pepper, etc.

Tip: **Warm or hot spices, which raise *yang*, are recommended for a vegetarian diet to balance the cooling effect of vegetable foods. Foods in general should be seasoned more strongly during cold months to prevent *yang* vacuity.**

Meal Preparation in Tune with the Five Phases (Wood, Fire, Earth, Metal, Water)

Cooking in tune with the five phases wood, fire, earth, metal, and water is a special method to harmoniously increase the energetic level of a dish. This cooking method follows the engendering (*sheng*) cycle.

The ingredients used in a dish are divided according to the phases they belong to, positioned in a row, and added to the dish in sequence. In keeping with the engendering cycle, the individual phases potentiate each other's energetic effect and increase the overall energetic aspect of the dish.

Practical Application:

- First, heat a pot on a heat source (fire phase). Add oil (earth phase) to move the cooking process one step further in the engendering cycle. To continue the cycle, follow earth with metal ingredients (e.g., onions). Next, add water ingredients (e.g., water with some salt). Now add wood foods (e.g., tomato). Next, add fire foods (e.g., thyme). This completes the first round of the engendering cycle.
- Now the cycle can begin again, starting with earth (e.g., carrots), followed by metal (e.g., leeks). Each complete cycle may be repeated as often as desired. The more often the cycle is run, the higher the energetic effect of the meal. Each of the phases should be allowed to influence the meal for at least half a minute before a new phase (ingredient) follows. No phase may be skipped within a cycle.
- Individual ingredients may be repeated as often as desired. For example, if using carrots as the only earth ingredient, some of the carrots can be added each time the earth phase comes up in a cycle. If more than one earth phase ingredient is used, carrots can be added in the first cycle, sweet potatoes in the second, and zucchini in the third.
- The phase used to end the Taoist cycle is discretionary, but the last phase added to the dish does impact the overall effect of the dish on the body. If the final ingredient is a pinch of salt, the overall energetic aspect of the meal is focused on the water phase (kidneys). If cooking concludes with a wood ingredient, for example vinegar, the dish will emphasize the wood phase (liver and gallbladder).

Seemingly strange and unusual ingredients that allow a continuation of the engendering cycle may have a surprisingly positive effect on the overall flavor of the meal.

2 Chinese Dietetics in Practice

Basic Recommendations of Chinese Dietetics

The Path to Healthy Eating Habits

Based on its observations and the experience of centuries, Chinese dietetics introduces a broad spectrum of valuable, practical recommendations for a healthy, holistic diet.

Along with the right choice of foods and preparation methods, Chinese nutrition also emphasizes healthy eating habits and developing a lifelong, healthy approach to food.

Inner Attitude and Environment

Eating with Enjoyment and in a Relaxed Atmosphere

Eating with delight and enjoyment in a leisurely and relaxed atmosphere and without any external distractions creates excellent conditions for good regeneration of *qi* from food. Positive feelings and moods generally promote good *qi* flow. During meals, positive feelings enable free flow of stomach and spleen *qi*, which supports the smooth processing of food and effective integration of food *qi* in the body.

Exhausting talks, discussions, and distractions (TV, radio, reading) burden stomach and spleen, which are especially sensitive to emotional tensions such as brooding, worries, anger, and fear. Negative emotions block and weaken the *qi* of digestive organs, resulting in loss of appetite, bloating, regurgitation, and stomach pain. "It turned my stomach"; "It ruined my appetite"; "The news made me choke on my food" are popular ways of describing this all too common situation.

Continuous exposure of the stomach/spleen network to emotional stress can cause serious eating disorders and digestive problems such as obesity, bulimia, anorexia, or gastric ulcers.

The classic texts recommend:
"When angry, it is easy to swallow food, but hard to digest it. When sad, it is hard to swallow and digest food. When experiencing strong emotions, it is advisable to delay eating until they have disappeared. Foods should always be ingested at the proper time. This makes it easier to digest them. Delaying eating and being able to digest food is better than eating too soon and not being able to digest. Digestive problems are accompanied by trouble, while good digestion frees a person from worry. It is not advisable to eat when strong emotions are brewing."

Well-chewed food supports spleen *qi*, satisfies hunger more quickly, and prevents obesity.

Tip: Chinese doctors recommend chewing each bite 10–15 times before swallowing. This prevents weight problems.

"*Stop when it tastes best*" is a good basic principle for determining the right amount to eat. Sleepiness or a burdened feeling should not appear after a meal. After excessively large meals, the entire *qi* and blood of the body is pulled into the center burner to cope with the excess. This initially results in bloating and drowsiness, and in case of protracted excess, weakens the digestive organs and causes dampness and phlegm disorders.

General Recommendations

Cooking Methods

Chinese dietetics recommends to **always** "unlock" all foods by using appropriate cooking methods to make them more accessible and digestible for the body. This protects center burner *qi* and allows for more effective transformation of food *qi*.

Tip: Grains, preferably freshly ground whole grains, always require cooking (boiling, simmering, steaming).

Traditional Chinese Medicine (TCM) recommends that raw foods, fruit, and especially tropical fruit should be used in moderation, contrary to some Western views. Except when part of specific healing diets or during the *yang* phase of summer, these foods are energetically too cool for most Northern latitudes and can cause long-term vacuity of the center burner when consumed in excess.

Common Syndromes
Spleen/pancreas *qi* vacuity, spleen/pancreas *yang* vacuity, phlegm disorders

Food Quantity

50–80%: Grains form the main share of a healthy diet in Chinese dietetics, for example corn, barley, millet, oats, rice, spelt, wheat
30–40%: Cooked vegetables, for example carrots, potatoes, fennel, beans, cabbage, legumes (beans and lentils).
5%: Meat, for example beef, lamb, game, also poultry, or even better fish, because it is easier to digest and develops less dampness.
5%: Raw foods, salads, fruit should make up only a small portion of the overall diet; more during the summer.
TCM recommends the intake of only small amounts of liquid (*yin*) during meals. Excess liquid drowns the stomach's digestive fire. The major share of the daily intake of liquids should be consumed between meals.

Food Quality

Fresh, unpolluted, naturally grown and produced foods are considered most valuable in TCM. Freshness is the highest priority, because fresh foods contain the most *qi* and optimally develop their specific thermal effect.
Industrial processing methods and most preservatives denature *qi*, which degrades food quality. In Chinese dietetics, such foods have weak or empty *qi* and are energetically inferior.

Avoid:
- Polluted foods
- Innards
- Highly processed and denatured foods
- Food additives
- Refined sugar and sweeteners
- Frozen foods
- Microwaving

Tip: Refined sugar should be substituted with natural sweeteners, such as raw cane sugar (e.g., Rapadura, an unrefined sugar made from whole raw sugar cane), honey, maple syrup, pear syrup, molasses made from sugar cane, apple butter, or palm sugar.

Flavor

The body's "inner voice" often reveals instinctively which flavor is of special significance. As part of a balanced lifestyle, one may give in to this inclination without hesitation.

Example
Craving sweets makes sense during exhausting mental work or strong physical exertion, since the sweet flavor has the strongest supplementing effect and most quickly regenerates *qi*. However, obvious, one-sided preference for a single flavor over a longer period is a diagnostic indicator for a potential imbalance. If a patient, for example, over months or even years seems to prefer sweet flavors, this may indicate disharmony of the earth phase reflecting an underlying disorder of the stomach, spleen/pancreas organ network.

Energetic Thermal Quality

Foods with a balanced thermal nature should be given preference in the daily diet: neutral, warm, or cool, depending on the times of day, seasons, bioclimatic factors, and constitution.
Acrid, warming spices and herbs may be used generously to support the stomach, spleen/pancreas network in its digestive function. Combining energetically cold and cool foods with warming foods is very beneficial, for example tomato salad with feta cheese, hot peppers, and garlic.
Hot and cold foods are thermal extremes and are employed rather sparingly, unless they are used to specifically treat beginning or established patterns of disharmony.

Example

Sudden change in weather, pathogenic factor wind-cold

Symptoms

Beginning cold with shivering, aversion to cold, sneezing. Cold extremities require *yang* energy to defend against external pathogenic cold and transport defense *qi* to the surface.

Nutritional Therapy

Acrid spices such as ginger, garlic, chili, cinnamon, pepper, hot tea with spices, mulled wine, and acridly seasoned soups make sense during such times.

Excessive use of the two energetic extremes hot and cold is not recommended, since they can easily bring about pathological *yang* or *yin* patterns of disharmony.

Special Significance of the Earth Phase

"Strengthening the Inner Center"

The earth phase and the stomach and spleen/pancreas network (center burner) are of key significance in Chinese dietetics.

Earth is *yin*, nourishing the core, inner balance, stability, and inner center. The center burner nourishes *yin*. It develops acquired constitution *qi* and *yang* and is responsible for intake, processing, and digestion of foods. According to TCM, a large part (about 70%) of the postnatal, renewable *qi* is taken from *gu qi* (drum *qi*).

Li Gao, the famous Chinese scholar of the *Song* dynasty (AD 960–1280), emphasized the special status of the center burner by founding a school just for the "strengthening of the center," which specifically focused on prevention, diagnosis, and therapy of the center burner.

During the Ming Dynasty (AD 1368–1644), the following quote developed: "Knowing how to treat the center is knowing how to bring all networks into balance."

All therapy began with "strengthening the inner center," the consistent development and protection of the stomach and spleen/pancreas network, primarily through nutritional therapy.

Many doctors were of the opinion that only when the Center Burner is balanced can the body form enough *qi*, blood, and body fluids. This forms the basis for subsequent therapies such as acupuncture.

The physician Sun Si Miao said this in the classical texts: "When treating an illness, the first step should be dietary therapy. Only when this is unsuccessful should one try drugs," and further, "Without knowledge of a proper diet it is hardly possible to enjoy good health."

This once again illustrates the importance of strengthening the function of the center burner daily through appropriate diet, in order to build up enough food *qi* to optimally regenerate the body's entire acquired *qi*.

If this network is weakened (stomach *qi* vacuity or spleen/pancreas *qi* or *yang* vacuity), the body invariably develops acute and later chronic *qi* or *yang* vacuity.

For daily strengthening of stomach and spleen *qi* and *yang*, warm and neutral foods from the earth phase with sweet flavor and upbearing movement are generally the most appropriate.

Foods that Strengthen the Center Burner
Foods from the Earth Phase
Grains
Millet Corn Oats Rice
Vegetables
Carrots Cabbage (all types) Fennel Potatoes Peas Squash, pumpkin Soy beans
Meat
Beef, veal Poultry, duck, goose Lamb, goat Venison Fish Bass Carp Herring Mackerel Sardine
Raw foods
Sweet apples Dates, figs Grapes Papaya
Beverages
Fennel tea (especially for infants and children) Grape juice Liqueurs

Tip: **Aperitifs or herbal liqueurs (e.g., aniseed or star anise) with warming effect of high-proof alcoholic beverages and warming herbs, before or after meals, are supportive "medicine" for the stomach and spleen/pancreas network.**

While the spleen is responsible for the production of *qi*, the stomach is responsible for the production of body fluids. The stomach should be supported with moistening, cooling foods that have a downbearing movement.

Avoid:

- Foods with cool and cold thermal nature; too many raw foods, citrus fruits, salad, or fruit. They cool down the body too much and weaken *qi* and *yang*, especially stomach and spleen *qi*.
- An excess of dairy products; they are energetically cool and cause dampness and phlegm.
- An excess of sweet, "heavy," or fatty foods; they weaken spleen *qi* and form dampness and phlegm.

! Foods that are energetically too cool, as well as refrigerated foods, significantly cool down the stomach's digestive fire. Cold blocks *qi* flow and causes food stagnation, resulting in stomach *qi* ascending counterflow. *Symptoms*: Nausea, vomiting, bloating, and gas. Acute and especially protracted use of foods that are too "cold" weaken stomach and spleen *qi* and *yang* permanently, with symptoms such as loss of appetite, chronic fatigue, sloppy stool, slight shivering, cold hands and feet.

In case of "chronic cooling" of the center burner (an excess of dairy or raw foods), the lower burner is forced to produce more warmth. Protracted exposure can weaken kidney fire and cause kidney *yang* vacuity.

Foods to Support Spleen *Yang*:	**Foods to Support Stomach *Yin*:**
Bass, beef, carrots, all cabbage varieties, crayfish, corn, fennel, potatoes, poultry, oats, soy beans, venison	All cabbage varieties, cheese, duck, eggplant, goose, milk, pork, potatoes, rice, tofu, tomatoes, wheat

Nutrition and Daily Rhythms

The classic texts recommend:
"Meals should always be taken at the proper time. This makes them easier to digest," and further, "Yang qi increases around noon and is weak at sunset. Thus eat a hearty breakfast, a small lunch, and a frugal meal in the evening and at night."

The following three main meals should be eaten daily and at about the same time, when possible supplemented by two smaller meals (snacks), for example around 11 a.m. and 4 p.m.

Breakfast

Since the stomach is at its optimal digestive capacity between 7 and 9 a.m., the morning meal should be substantial and fortifying.
A good breakfast strengthens stomach and spleen *qi* and *yang* for the day. Optimal breakfast foods are energetically warming foods, prepared with warm cooking methods that stimulate the body and do not spread dampness.

Recommended

An ideal start to a good day begins with a cooked (warm) porridge of grains, ideally freshly ground, especially millet, corn, or the very warming oats (e.g., oatmeal). During summer, the slightly cooler wheat is recommended. The porridge can be combined with nuts, seeds, and a little seasonal fruit. If needed, sweeten lightly to supplement, using honey or marmalade or the other sweeteners mentioned earlier. Black tea or coffee, both in moderation, are suitable breakfast beverages to support *yang*.

Avoid

Energetically cold and dampness-producing foods that suppress the expanding morning *yang* and weaken digestive fire, i.e., fruit, fruit juices, raw foods, excess dairy products.

Note: Dairy products are appropriate in small amounts when spleen qi is good. Otherwise, they are energetically too cold and can easily cause dampness or phlegm.

Lunch

Lunch is preferably a substantial, warm meal that strengthens the center burner. Warming grains and vegetables are highly recommended, as well as fish, poultry, some lean meat and salad.

> ***Tip:*** **A good meal does not burden the body or cause drowsiness. Avoid fatty, oily foods, foods that are too cold, or meals that are too big. They produce dampness in the body, slow down *qi* flow, and cause fatigue and sluggishness.**

Evening Meal/Dinner

In the evening, *yang* and digestive capacity decrease and *yin* increases. The evening meal should be small and support the growing *yin*, for example warm grain and vegetable dishes, possibly some meat, moderate amounts of dairy or soy products and a small amount of beer.

Avoid:

Energetically hot, stimulating foods, such as acridly seasoned foods.

> ***Tip:*** Opulent meals in the evening burden the stomach and spleen *qi*, which is naturally lower in the evening. Often, such meals result in weight gain, nausea, bloating, and disturbed sleep. People with weight problems should not eat at all after 6 p.m., when digestive organs are at their weakest.

Nutrition and Seasonal Rhythms

A multitude of the body's internal processes follow natural external changes of the seasons. By developing eating habits and choosing foods that are in tune with the seasons, we can integrate ourselves into these rhythms in a natural way. Chinese dietetics views this as beneficial for promoting natural *qi* flow, compensating for weather effects and preventing potential development of disorders.

> **Tip:** Choosing foods that are local and in season is good and easy advice to follow.

Spring

Spring is the season of the beginning small *yang* and is characterized by growth, movement, and expansion. The body's *qi* flows strongly again and seeks to expand freely. Food during this season should supplement *qi*, allow it to course freely, and support spleen and liver functions.

Recommended Spring Foods

- Mildly warming foods with upbearing movement: Fennel, rice, buckwheat; possibly acrid flavors (garlic, paprika, ginger) in case of accumulated dampness left over from the colder months.
- Sour flavors, because they stabilize liver *yin* and can regulate upbearing liver *yang*.
- Foods from the wood phase, green in color with neutral, cool, or warm energy: Green tea, spinach, celery, a little more raw foods and sprouts

Wind is often the dominating weather effect during spring and causes recurring external wind disorders (colds, flu), which can be balanced with the mildly acrid flavors of green onions and ginger.

Avoid:

Energetically hot and fatty foods, as they block liver *qi*, and excess sour flavors.

Summer (Hot Season)

Summer is the season of the big *yang* and is characterized by the fire phase and summer heat. Heat feeds on body fluids and harms *yin*. It is recommended to take in predominately cooling, dampness-providing foods (*yin* food) to disperse heat and build up body fluids. The bitter flavor corresponds to the fire phase, and mostly bitter–cool as well as bitter–cold foods in moderation should be consumed during the hot season.

Recommended Summer Foods

- Fruit or fruit juices: Apple, lemon, kiwi, melon, orange, pear, pineapple, tangerine
- *Cooling foods*: Cucumber, Belgian endive hearts, spinach, tomato, as well as more raw foods, salads, yogurt, wheat, barley, black or even better green tea, mineral water, wheat beer, mussels, rabbit

> **Tip:** The Chinese have recommended green tea as an ideal beverage during summer heat for centuries. *"It disperses summer heat and can expel toxins, cool the heart fire, calm the mind, remove heat from liver and gallbladder, and relieve stomach and lung."*

Avoid:

Dry and energetically hot foods such as coffee (!) and acrid spices. Also avoid ice-cold foods and beverages and ice cream, because they abruptly block the stomach's digestive energy.

In the view of Chinese medicine, children have a physiologically weak center burner until they are about eight years old. They are especially sensitive to cold foods and beverages.

Symptoms

Sudden diarrhea and vomiting, often in the summer after extensive swimming (external cold), in combination with ice cream and cold beverages.

Nutritional Therapy

Fennel tea with spices

Autumn

Autumn is characterized by the external decline of nature and, in many climates, by drying and cooling. The natural movement pattern of autumn is directed inward. *Yang* energy decreases, the small *yin* appears, and the energies of the body gather on the inside. Foods with downbearing movement and sour flavor (apple) support "inner" composure and serenity in the body.

Recommended Autumn Foods

Mildly acrid and energetically warm foods that compensate for the onset of external cold such as oats, millet, corn, rice, carrots, leeks, radishes, cauliflower, beef, lamb. For inner cold, shivering, and the beginning of a cold, the acrid flavors of garlic, cinnamon, chili, ginger, and onions stimulate *qi* circulation and rapidly bring defensive energy to the surface.

For external dampness, warm, dry foods should be used to support the center burner (millet, rice) and the lungs (acrid spices to drive away dampness and phlegm disorders). If dryness predominates, moistening foods (pear, tofu, peanuts) should be utilized.

Avoid:

Fatty, oily foods, and cool or cold dairy products, which burden the spleen and cause dampness and phlegm disorders (bronchitis, sinusitis), especially during wet weather (see "Dampness and Phlegm Disorders," p. 64).

Winter (Cold Season)

Winter is the period when the big *yin* gathers and hides *qi* in deeper layers, which makes the body more susceptible to cold disorders. During the colder months, a warm, supplementing diet with acrid and sweet flavors that builds up and moves *qi* and protects it against cold stagnations is important.

Recommended Winter Foods

Warm meats that supplement qi, yang and blood: Lamb, venison, game, beef, poultry, duck, stews with legumes and meat; also grapes and red wine.

The cold season diet should focus on strengthening kidney and spleen *yang* with lamb, venison, prawns, high-proof alcoholic beverages, acrid spices, aniseed (star anise), cloves, tea with spices, fennel, leek, walnuts, chestnuts, black sesame, oysters.

The best time to build up *qi* and blood with a sweet, supplementing diet is at the end of winter.

Li Shi Chin, at the time of the Ming Dynasty, recommends moderate, but regular consumption of alcohol. "Alcoholic beverages are bitter and acrid in flavor and hot in thermal nature. When consumed regularly and in the right amount, alcohol regulates blood flow, promotes qi circulation, stimulates the mind, and warms the body."

! A word of caution: "All good things in moderation ..."

Avoid:

An excess of energetically hot, warm, and acrid foods because they dry up body fluids, weaken *yin*, and encourage *yang* repletion disorders.

Nutrition and Pathogenic Factors

The pathogenic factors heat, cold, dampness, dryness, and wind have a significant effect on the body. Nutritional therapy can remove the damaging effects of external climate factors, as well as internal pathological states. Sudden weather changes often require rapid and flexible changes in diet.

Cold

When the body is affected by cold, it should be supplied with sufficient *yang* energy with the help of energetically hot and warm food. The acrid-spicy and sweet flavors, as well as hearty dishes, should be favored.

Nutritional Therapy
Acrid spices such as chili, ginger, cinnamon, garlic, star anise, cloves, onions, Chinese leeks (garlic chives), coriander.
Also high-proof alcoholic beverages, mulled wine, grog (a hot rum beverage with spices similar to hot buttered rum), cooking with alcohol, tea with spices, oats, fennel, lamb, venison.

Heat

Heat calls for energetically cooling and cold foods, as well as the bitter and sour flavors. For dehydration and external dryness, foods should also moisten.

Nutritional Therapy
Cooling fruit such as pineapple, tangerine, melon, orange, lemon, kiwi. Cooling vegetables such as dandelion, tomato, cucumber, Belgian endive hearts, spinach.
Also salads, mung bean sprouts, yogurt, wheat, barley, black or better green tea, mineral water, wheat beer.

Dampness

Dampness calls for warming, drying, and dampness-transforming foods, because they supplement the spleen. Bitter-warm flavors, warm-sweet flavors and warm-acrid flavors should be preferred.

Nutritional Therapy
Millet, rice, amaranth, pear, cherries, grapes, and warming spices like ginger (in moderation).

Avoid:
Oily, fatty foods, excessively sweet foods, fatty meats, pork, bananas, sugar, too much dairy.

Note: Protracted dampness can cause phlegm. This calls for dry foods, such as millet or Belgian endive hearts, and bitter-warm, sweet-neutral, or sweet-warm flavors. Moderately acrid flavors can dissolve phlegm stagnation. With phlegm disorders, fatty-oily foods should be avoided, as should foods that are too hot. Consumption of phlegm-producing foods, such as dairy products and banana, should also be reduced.

Dryness

Dryness calls for fluid-promoting, moistening foods, refreshing vegetables, fruit and vegetable juices, as well as salads.

Nutritional Therapy
Pear, melon, tomato, banana, grapes, wheat, peanuts, pine nuts, soy products, dairy products, pork.

External Wind

External wind often acts as a carrier for the weather factors cold and heat.

Wind–Cold

Nutritional Therapy

Acrid spices such as chili, ginger, cinnamon, garlic, green onions.

Wind–Heat

Nutritional Therapy

Eggplant, green tea, watermelon, chamomile tea.

Internal Wind

Internal wind has a distinct *yang* character: Dizziness, tremors, spasms, disturbed vision.

Nutritional Therapy

Avoid all foods that move *qi*.

Preferable: Eggplant, celery, water chestnut, sunflower seeds, banana, pike/perch, bass, rabbit.

Nutrition and the Human Life Cycle

Children and Young People

Children should be introduced to good eating habits early. A healthy diet that develops body and mind is of vital importance to their health later in life. Strengthening the center burner is a priority, since it is still underdeveloped in children. Neutral to mildly warming foods of the sweet flavor are ideal for children.

Nutritional Therapy for Children
Millet, rice, barley, carrots, fennel, apples, honey, raisins, poultry, beef, potatoes, grape juice, fennel tea.
Children have a natural craving for sweet foods and require "sweet" in the view of TCM, because it is the best flavor for strengthening the center burner.

Tip: Sugar should be replaced with natural sweeteners such as honey, maple syrup, pear juice, molasses from sugar cane, apple butter, and sweet, warming fruits. Popular and ideal for kids are raisins and dates, displayed in a visually appealing way.

Avoid:
Energetically cold, cool foods, acrid spices, sugar, excess dairy products, fatty foods.
A healing diet is well-suited for treating children with already manifest disorders (hyperactivity, allergies, headaches) and is well tolerated. Often, reduced intake of specific foods or substances and a change of diet is all that is needed for lasting improvements in children. Nutritional therapy is also important for children when combined with other methods of healing.

Midlife

During the middle phase of life, generally all foods are suitable. The diet should be varied and in tune with individual constitution, the seasons, and the weather. General nutritional guidelines should be followed.

Avoid:
An unbalanced diet and an excess of meat, raw foods, fats, dairy products, and coffee.

Older People

Several smaller meals throughout the day are recommended for older people, since their digestive fire is weaker and meals can be more easily digested that way. Diet should prevent *qi* or blood vacuity. Center burner and kidney essence should be supported.

Preferred Foods for Older People
Well cooked foods, porridge, eggs, fish, stews, Master Soups.

Avoid:
Raw foods, fatty, oily, or roasted dishes, excessive salt consumption.

3 Practical Application of Chinese Dietetics

A General Applications of Chinese Dietetics

Practical Guidelines for Giving Nutritional Advice

The Role of Chinese Nutrition in Traditional Chinese Medicine (TCM)

Nutrition has played an important role in China's traditional medical system for many centuries and continues to do so. Chinese physicians have always regarded food as medicine. Eating a balanced diet was how the body was kept in harmony. Changing weather conditions throughout the year were taken into account by adjusting the diet accordingly and choosing the appropriate ingredients.
Today, nutrition is still firmly rooted in public awareness in China and is regarded as an essential element in achieving a long and fulfilled life. The Chinese diet is a preventive diet. External climate factors determine daily food choices. In times of extreme cold, dishes using acrid spices provide increased nourishment for the body. In winter, the emphasis is on warming and hot dishes, while in times of extreme external heat, the body is calmed with cooling dishes. Such a preventive diet can be practiced in other parts of the world and can be followed by most people. It requires no special expertise other than a general understanding of Chinese nutritional principles. Healing diets that address imbalance, however, require a clear diagnosis and development of a therapy strategy by a professional TCM practitioner.

General Indications for Chinese Dietetics

- Daily general regeneration and balancing of *qi*, blood (*xue*), body fluids (*jin ye*), and spirit (*shen*).
- Specific supplementation of *qi*, *yang*, *yin*, and especially blood (*xue*) and body fluids (*jin ye*).
- Stabilizing, invigorating, or calming the spirit (*shen*).
- Preserving essence (*jing*) with high-quality foods and regular eating habits.
- Supplementing and balancing the organ networks and the bowels and viscera (*zang fu* organs).
- Supplementing, regenerating, and moving defense *qi* (*wei qi*).
- Supplementing and balancing the spleen/pancreas and stomach organ networks.
- Balancing disturbing effects brought on by weather or other external factors.
- Harmonizing the body with the seasons.

In essence, diet influences all functions and processes in the body.
A few other proven indications for Chinese nutrition should also be mentioned here:

- Supplementing the center burner in children.
- Treating patterns of disharmony in children.
- Prevention during pregnancy by strengthening *qi*, particularly blood (*xue*) and body fluids (*jin yc*).
- General regeneration after childbirth, especially in cases of exhaustion.
- Specific treatment of constitutional disorders.
- Treating disorders caused by dampness and phlegm.

- Treating acute and chronic conditions. This includes disorders of the respiratory system, allergies, acute and chronic gastrointestinal disorders, skin disorders, gynecological disorders, menopausal symptoms, urological disorders, insomnia, psychological instabilities, exhaustion, weight gain, hyperactivity.

Don't Worry about Dogmatism

Chinese nutrition has nothing to do with rigid diets or instructions that have to be followed dogmatically. On the contrary, enjoyment involving all the senses is a vital part of any diet. Nor does it mean that from now on all one's meals have to be eaten with chopsticks, or that the fridge has to be stocked with bamboo sprouts, Chinese (napa) cabbage, and tofu. The principles of Chinese nutrition can be applied to any cuisine or cooking style. The only knowledge that is required is an understanding of the thermal and energetic principles of foods, spices, and cooking methods, and an awareness of the adjustments to be made for seasons, climate effects, physical constitution, and individual sensitivities.

Tips for Giving Nutritional Advice

Basic knowledge of Chinese nutrition enables anyone to manage their health by choosing the right foods and developing healthy eating habits. This primarily requires a knowledge of the thermal nature of foods (see the tables at the back of this book, p. 220) to respond appropriately to seasonal changes, climate factors such as cold, dampness, and summer heat, or extreme physical or emotional strain.

However, people new to TCM, even when in good health, quickly start asking questions about their own constitution, individual food choices, different interactions, dietary habits, etc.

People interested in prevention through diet can benefit from consulting a qualified TCM practitioner who can give specific advice. The confidence a practitioner can instill for the individualized application of Chinese nutrition at home makes such a consultation a worthwhile investment.

Important: Nutritional therapy designed to heal illness must always be based on an informed diagnosis by a qualified TCM practitioner. Therapy must consider both the possibilities and the limitations of nutritional healing. Dietary therapy is commonly used in conjunction with other methods of Chinese medicine. Experienced TCM practitioners can also achieve excellent results by combining TCM with the diagnosis and therapy of Western medicine and naturopathy—all to the patient's advantage.

The following tips help you achieve compliance in your patients, which is so crucial to the success of dietary advice!

When prescribing a preventive diet, acknowledge your patients' individual preferences to achieve the greatest possible compliance.

In cases where a healing diet is appropriate, a patient's distinct preferences can provide valuable therapeutic clues to patterns of disharmony.

A patient's constitution should be at the center of any decisions made about dietary prescriptions.

Dietary recommendations always need to be adapted to the seasons and bioclimatic factors.

Chinese nutrition requires more time than other treatments and thus a little patience. Let your patients know that tangible results might not be felt or seen for weeks or months, but that, once achieved, these results can last a lifetime. Inform your patients that dietary therapy is a great opportunity for developing healthy and beneficial eating habits that will keep them in good health for years to come.

Suggestions for giving dietary advice

- To give competent and professional dietary advice, you should have a sound knowledge of the principles of Chinese nutrition (both preventive and healing diets) and should be trained in TCM diagnosis.
- During the initial consultation, you can assess your patient's constitution by paying attention to certain criteria and then deepen your observations by asking your patient specific questions.
- Let your patients tell you about their eating habits, food preferences, etc.
- Ask your patients about their digestion.
- Communicate the results of your observations to your patients and explain in detail the diet plan that will accompany them in the following weeks.
- Clearly mark all foods that are good for the patient with a "+," and foods that are bad for the patient with a "–";
- Make recommendations about eating habits and food preparation (tailored to the diagnosis) during the initial consultation.
- Provide your patient with written information. This includes:
  - An individual diet plan with a list of all foods that are appropriate for the patient;
  - General basic information about energetic principles, healthy eating habits, different cooking methods, supplementing the center burner, etc.
  - Copies of recipes for specific preparations, such as the Master Soup, congees, medicinal wines (see p. 33, 117, 160).

This makes your own work easier, takes less time, and enables patients to explore the information at their own pace at home.

- Length of initial consultation: between 20 and 100 minutes.
- Arrange a second appointment three to six weeks later.
- Possible follow-up questions can be answered over the phone (have a phone consultation schedule).
- During the second consultation, answer any questions and clear up any uncertainties. Have the patient describe any noticeable successes or results.

General Nutritional Recommendations (for sharing with patients)

Please take the following to heart:

- Use high-quality, clean, and unprocessed foods, organically grown whenever possible.
- Create a pleasant, relaxed atmosphere in which you can enjoy your meals.
- Eat with pleasure.
- Eat regularly, between three to five times a day.
- Do not rush your meals and chew each bite well (between 10 and 15 times)!
- Eat breakfast like a king, lunch like an emperor, and dinner like a beggar.
- Stop eating when it tastes best!
- Drink only small amounts of liquids during meals; too much liquid with meals, or right before and right after a meal can weaken your digestive fire.
- When putting together a meal, take into account your individual constitution.
- Choose foods that are appropriate for the season (choosing locally grown foods that are in season is often a good way).
- When following a vegetarian diet, ensure your diet contains enough energetically warming foods; increase the use of acrid spices in cold weather.

Please avoid the following:

- *Too much raw or cold food and tropical fruits*: These are energetically too cool, reduce the energy of the center burner, and if consumed, regularly, can cool the kidney organ network.
- *Ice-cold beverages*: They block stomach and spleen/pancreas *qi* flow and weaken spleen *qi* and spleen *yang*.
- *Too much dairy*: Dairy products are energetically too cool. They weaken the spleen/pancreas network and cause dampness and phlegm.
- Exhausting discussions or other distractions during a meal (TV, radio, reading): They can block the flow of qi in the center burner and cause food stagnation.
- *Too much oily, fatty food*: Blocks the flow of *qi* and causes heat, dampness, and phlegm.
- *Too much sugar, sweet flavors*: Causes heat, dampness and phlegm.
- *Too much alcohol*: Causes damp heat, promotes formation of phlegm and hurts *jing*, along with a number of other unpleasant effects.
- *Too much meat:* Causes dampness and phlegm.
- *Late evening meals*: Block the flow of *qi*, cause food obstruction, weaken the spleen/pancreas network, and lead to weight gain.
- *Overly opulent meals*: Block flow of *qi*, cause food stagnation, burden the spleen/pancreas network, cause dampness and phlegm and lead to weight gain.
- *Excessive and prolonged fasting*: Weakens the center burner, as well as *yin*, blood (*xue*), and *jing*.

Application Areas

Application Goal: Prevention

The main application for Chinese nutrition is prevention and general healthy living. Mild states of disharmony that are common in everyday life, for example those caused by bioclimatic factors such as cold or heat, or brought on by times of stress, can be balanced with appropriate preparation and choice of foods. Choosing foods in accordance and harmony with the seasons protects the body against disorders and helps it to live in tune with natural rhythms.

Example

During the cold seasons (fall and winter in the Northern hemisphere), one should increase the intake of warm or hot foods with pronounced *yang* character. Fruits and salads—foods that are mostly *yin*—are not recommended during the colder months, because they cool down the energetics of the body even further, instead of warming it and protecting it from external cold.

Application Goal: Therapy

Therapy always first requires a diagnosis based on the principles of TCM. The appropriate choice of foods provides a foundation for further treatment methods such as acupuncture and herbal therapy. Dietary therapy adjusted to the individual's symptoms creates a good basis for additional treatments, resulting in quicker and more effective improvement. Chinese practitioners find it hard to understand why most doctors in the Western world utilize only one treatment at a time, for example acupuncture, instead of making full use of all treatments available and coming up with a comprehensive treatment strategy. In traditional Chinese hospitals, a patient's individual diet plan is part of a holistic treatment concept.

Example

The treatment of insomnia, which aims to drain *yang*, will not prove successful through acupuncture alone if patients continue to stimulate their *yang* by consuming warm or hot foods. Examples are coffee, hot spices, garlic, onions, and lamb. By ignoring dietary recommendations, the patient essentially works against the acupuncture treatment rather than with it. Abstaining from foods containing *yang* and giving preference to *yin* foods, on the other hand, supports the acupuncture treatment and promotes success.

General *Qi* Vacuity

Qi vacuity can appear in any of the networks. The most common causes for general *qi* vacuity are vacuity of spleen *qi*, kidney *qi*, and lung *qi*.

Symptoms

Fatigue, exhaustion, lack of appetite, lack of concentration, abdominal bloating; soft, sloppy stool; tendency to diarrhea, tendency to feel cold and to shiver, aversion to cold, lowered resistance, frequent backaches in the lumbar vertebral column, frequent urination with clear urine, large amounts of urine, nocturia (excessive night time urination), dyspnea (shortness of breath), premature ejaculation, reduced sexual desire, impotence.

Tongue: Pale, swollen

Pulse: Vacuous, weak

Causes

General: Stress, overexertion, lack of sleep, too many negative emotions such as worries, anxiety, fear, brooding; too much sexual activity; in women, too many births spaced too closely; external cold; chronic illnesses.

Diet: Too much thermally cold food, *yin* products, or raw foods; irregular eating habits; too much dairy; too many tropical fruits, frozen foods, denaturalized foods, canned foods, or ice-cold beverages; hasty eating; eating too late in the day.

Prevention

Nutritional Therapy

Thermal nature	Neutral, warming, sometimes hot
Cooking method	Warming
Flavor	Neutral–sweet, warm–sweet, neutral–acrid, warm–acrid, neutral–salty, warm–salty, occasionally also hot
Grains	Oats, millet, corn, rice, short-grain (sweet, glutinous) rice, spelt
Meat	Poultry, lamb, beef, game (venison)
Fish	Oysters, trout, lobster, salmon, anchovies
Vegetables	Fennel, carrots, leeks, chestnuts
Spices	Acrid and hot, ginger, garlic, coriander
Nuts and seeds	Hazelnuts, black sesame, walnuts
Legumes	Lentils

Tip: Have a substantial, warming breakfast, for example warm millet porridge or oatmeal, and at least one or two warm meals daily, for example Master Soup, stews.

Supplement spleen *qi*

激 • ST-36 • CV-12 • SP-3

Supplement kidney *qi*

激 • CV- 6 • KI- 7 • Moxa

General *Yang* Vacuity

Yang vacuity can present similar symptoms as *qi* vacuity, because *yang* vacuity is always preceded by protracted *qi* vacuity and the transition between the two is not clearly delineated.

Symptoms

Primarily cold symptoms, such as cold, pale extremities, general weakness, severe mental and physical exhaustion, lack of drive, general loss of strength, as well as water retention in form of edemas. Women can encounter menstrual disorders, missed periods, and diarrhea.

Tongue: Pale, swollen, with tooth impressions
Pulse: Vacuous, weak

Prevention

Basically the same as for *qi* vacuity. However, more foods with strong *yang* character can be used.

Cooking method	Warming, grilled, fried
Meat	Beef, poultry, lamb, game (especially venison)
Also	Fennel, walnuts, chestnuts, corn, raisins, cherries, peaches, leeks, acrid spices

***Master** Soup and stews with warming meat and vegetables.*

Supplement kidney *yang*
激 • KI-7 • SP-3 • CV-6

Supplement spleen *yang*
激 • ST-36 + Moxa • GV-4 + Moxa

General *Yin* Vacuity

Yin vacuity is a deeper disorder of the body and can affect each of the organ networks. Syndromes seen frequently in practice are *yin* vacuity of the liver, heart, lung, and kidney networks. *Yin* vacuity can damage the substance of the organ network involved.

Symptoms

Thirst, dry mouth, hot soles of the feet, especially at night, possibly hot hands, burning sensation behind the chest bone, night sweat, possibly weight loss. *Symptoms that occur due to pseudo-yang as a result of yin vacuity*: Restlessness, agitation, nervousness, sleep disorders, dizziness, internal heat sensation; dry, hard stool; easily startled, emotional instability, susceptibility to stress, lack of resiliency.

Tongue: Red, chapped
Pulse: Rapid, thin.

Causes

General causes: Long chronic illnesses, depletion of body fluids, for example due to extreme fever; protracted blood loss; excessive sexual activity; excessive drug use or medication abuse; extreme emotional strain such as worry, grief, fear; overexertion and overwork; sleep deprivation due to nighttime work; hectic and stressful lifestyle that creates internal heat and exhausts body fluids.

Dietary causes: Excessive intake of extremely warming foods, especially acrid spices that dry out the body fluids and hurt the *yin*. Additional factors are excessive intake of coffee, high-proof alcoholic beverages, poor and irregular diet.

Prevention

Nutritional Therapy

Avoid:
Heat; foods with *yang* characteristics; the flavors hot–bitter, warm–bitter, hot–acrid, warm– acrid; hot and warm foods or beverages, especially coffee, black tea, red wine; garlic, ginger, acrid spices; high-proof alcohol.

Recommended:
Yin foods with neutral-sweet and refreshing-sweet flavor.

Meat/fish	Pork, oysters
Vegetables	Cooling, refreshing vegetables, spinach, tomatoes, seaweed
Grains	Spelt, corn, rice, wheat
Fruit	Apples, pears, blackberries, citrus fruit, strawberries, bananas, grapes
Dairy products	Butter, cheese, yogurt, milk
Soy products	Tofu, soy milk
Beverages	Red fruit juices, citrus juices, wheat beer

Replenish *yin* by supplementing spleen *yin*, kidney *yin*, and liver *yin*

激 • KI-3 • SP-6 • KI-6

激 • CV-6 • LR-8

Yin Repletion (Excess) and Dampness

Yin repletion is often caused by a poor, insufficient diet. Consuming too many *yin* products cools the body, harms spleen *qi*, and causes dampness. This syndrome can worsen due to a weak spleen and can, over time, lead to phlegm disorders. *Yin* repletion reduces the body's *yang* energy.

Symptoms
Lack of drive; fatigue; slowed movements and language; cold hands; feeling of heaviness inside the body, as well as in the arms and legs; dull headache which the patient often describes as a "feeling like I am wearing a helmet"; tendency to diarrhea, bloating, water retention in arms, legs, and face; a melancholic disposition, sometimes depression; obesity.

Causes
General causes: General factors that can cause spleen *qi* vacuity and general *yang* vacuity, such as overexertion, lack of sleep.
Dietary causes: Irregular intake of food; rushed meals eaten under stress; main meal in the late evening; too much raw food, salads and dairy products that produce too much dampness and phlegm.

Prevention

Successfully dealing with the stresses and challenges of everyday life while staying healthy requires a healthy and supportive diet. Healthy eating habits should be developed to sustain the energy necessary for facing the demands of daily life and establishing a balanced state of health.

Avoid:
Yin foods; damp foods, especially dairy products; raw fruit and vegetables; excess sweet flavors; hasty, irregular meals; main meal in the late evening; inadequate breakfast; too much fat and oil.

Recommended:
Moderately warming foods and cooking methods. For dampness and phlegm, especially bitter-warm flavors, but also sweet- warm, warm-salty, warm-refreshing, as well as all neutral flavors. Moderate intake of hot foods.
Also: Ginger, cardamom, leeks, pears, cherries, carp, millet.
For additional recommendations, see also "Strengthening the Inner Center," page 42.

Yang Repletion (Excess) Conditions

Yang repletion displays different levels of intensity and is a commonly found pattern of disharmony in medical practice. It is important to differentiate real *yang* repletion from "pseudo-*yang*" repletion or "*empty heat*." Real *yang* repletion is a short-term surplus of *yang*. "Pseudo-*yang*" repletion is the appearance of *yang* repletion symptoms caused by the absence of *yin*, which can lead to an increased appearance of *yang* character.
Draining *yang* can initially alleviate both patterns. If the cause is complete *yin* vacuity, as is the case

with "pseudo-*yang*" repletion, *yin* needs to be replenished along with draining *yang* in order to establish lasting harmony.

Symptoms

Red complexion, hyperactivity, restlessness, anxiety, loud voice, boisterous laugh, dominating personality, irritability, and tendency to outbursts of anger. Body feels hot, thirst, tendency to get headaches, dizziness, tinnitus (ringing in the ears), headache in the temporal region (*shao yang* headache due to upbearing liver *yang*), bitter taste in mouth (liver fire), excessive perspiration, high blood pressure, episodes of voracious appetite with a tendency to weight gain (stomach heat).

Causes

General causes: The majority of *yang* symptoms are caused by a relative *yang* surplus and result from a *yin* vacuity of the affected bowel (*zang* organ). Emotional strains such as stress, a hectic lifestyle, and suppressed emotions such as rage, anger, and frustration harm the organ network of heart and liver. The longer an emotional imbalance persists, the more the organs are impaired. The liver phase is especially sensitive and can suffer deep-seated damage from protracted stagnation of liver *qi* when *qi* flow is blocked due to suppressed emotions. This creates a precarious balance that can easily be upset by even minor *yang* effects such as stress or the wrong diet (high-proof alcohol, acrid spices), invoking symptoms of ascendant liver *yang* (*gan yang shang kang*) and liver fire (*gan huo shang yan*)

Dietary causes: Green tea, mineral water, wheat beer, tofu, mung beans, dandelion, Belgian endive hearts, peppermint tea, cow's milk, yogurt, cheese, farmer's cheese, cottage cheese, buttermilk.

Patients often prefer acrid flavors to relax the body and loosen any existing emotional blockages, or excessively sweet flavors to counteract frustrations and grief. Acrid–warm flavors and acrid–hot flavors, like all thermally hot foods, can cause heat-related symptoms. Bitter–hot, as well as all other hot flavors can dry out body fluids and deplete the body's *yin*. These heat symptoms often appear in combination with hot, viscous phlegm and frequently result from excessive consumption of very oily or fatty foods. The liver organ network is especially sensitive to heat and fatty, oily foods (junk food).

Prevention

Nutritional Therapy

Avoid:

All energetically hot foods and beverages, especially acrid spices such as curry, ginger, garlic, and pepper. Onions, high-proof alcohol, warming cooking methods like frying, grilling. Decrease consumption of thermally warm foods and meat (abstain from meat for four to six weeks, especially lamb, beef, poultry, pork). Decrease intake of coffee, red wine, and salt.

Recommended:

Yin foods with neutral–sweet, cool–sweet, cold–sweet, neutral–sour, cool–sour, cold–sour flavor.

Vegetables: Tomatoes, spinach, cucumbers, celery

Grains: Wheat, barley

Fruit: Apples, pears, citrus fruit, raspberries, gooseberries

■ Blood Vacuity (*Xue Xu*)

Blood vacuity is an important syndrome in Chinese pathophysiology and is very commonly found in practice. Blood vacuity is often at the root of many gynecological disorders. Men have more *qi* in their blood and thus tend to suffer more from *qi* problems.

Symptoms

General:	Pale skin, pale lips, sensation of dizziness inside head, dull complexion, numbness, fatigue, dry hair and skin.
Liver blood vacuity (gan xue xu):	Blurred vision, sleep disorders, dry and brittle nails, muscle weakness, muscle cramps, sensation of "pins and needles" or falling asleep of the limbs, sensitivity of eyes to light, psychological, mental, and gynecological symptoms, lack of drive, nervousness, emotional frailty, low self-esteem, heart palpitations, menstrual disorders such as painful menstruation or absence of menstruation (dysmenorrhea or amenorrhea).

Chronic blood vacuity symptoms are general dryness: Dry skin, dry hair, possibly hair loss, and brittle nails. Blood vacuity can create favorable conditions for liver wind, causing dry skin conditions accompanied by severe itching and blisters on alternating parts of the body.

Tongue: Pale, small; dry tongue body
Pulse: Thin, fine or rough

Pathogenesis

TCM believes that blood is primarily formed in the spleen. Blood vacuity can therefore be caused by spleen vacuity. Blood formed in the spleen with help from the lungs becomes "spirited" with *qi* and *jing* from the kidneys as it circulates. Not until then does blood from the spleen have the necessary energy. Good blood formation also requires balanced lung and kidney energy. The liver plays an important role as a storage organ for blood. This means that any blood vacuity eventually leads to liver disharmony with liver blood vacuity (*gan xue xu*). Particularly damaging to the blood is liver heat, which sets blood into restless motion. Protracted heat can dry out and damage blood (*xue*).

Therapy

Strengthen blood
Supplement spleen *qi*
Enrich liver blood

激 • SP-10 • ST-36 • BL-17 • SP-6 • LR-8 • SP-2 • BL-21

Nutritional Therapy

Avoid:

Warming cooking methods and thermally hot foods. All bitter foods, especially the flavors bitter–hot and bitter–warm. Acrid–hot and acrid–warm flavors, since these dry out blood. Black tea, hot chocolate, acrid spices such as garlic, ginger, pepper, curry, cinnamon, etc. Energetically hot drinks such as coffee, high-proof alcohol, yogi tea (chai).

Recommended:

Cooking method	Cooling
Flavor	Sweet–neutral, sweet–warm, sour–neutral, sour–cool
Grains	Oats, amaranth, short-grain (glutinous) rice, rice
Vegetables	All thermally neutral and refreshing vegetables like red beets, red cabbage, carrots, spinach, fennel
Meat	Chicken, chicken liver, beef, beef stock, beef liver, veal liver, lamb liver (liver preferably from organically raised animals or aninmals living in the wild)
Fish	Oysters, mussels, squid (octopus), perch, eel
Fruits	Red grapes, sweet cherries, longans (a type of lychee), plums, apricots
Nuts and seeds	Sesame, sunflower seeds
Beverages	Red beet juice, sweet cherry juice, plum juice, red tea (e.g., rosehip tea, hibiscus), red grape juice, red wine in moderation

Recommended for liver blood vacuity:

Meat	Chicken, duck, rabbit liver, hare liver, pork liver (liver preferably from organically raised or wild harvested animals)
Fish	Oysters, shrimps, white fish, bass
Fruit	Apples, lychees, plums, grapes, longans (similar to lychees)
Vegetables	Thermally neutral and cooling, green vegetables of the wood phase: beans, broccoli, lamb's lettuce (miner's lettuce), lotus root, mangold chard (Swiss chard), spinach, sprouts, tomatoes
Beverages	Carrot juice, tomato juice
Grains	Wheat, short-grain (glutinous) rice
Spices	Watercress, marjoram, parsley root
Nuts and seeds	Sesame, sunflower seeds
Other	Egg yolk

Strengthening Defense *Qi* (*Wei Qi*)

Defense *qi* protects the body against disease. It circulates outside the body channels, mainly on the body's surface. Defense *qi*'s most important function is to provide protection against external pathogenic factors such as wind, cold, heat, and dampness. At the same time, it warms and moistens skin and muscles. Since it circulates below the skin's surface, defense *qi* is primarily governed by the lungs. Defense *qi* prevents pathogens from entering the body by regulating the opening and closing of the skin's pores. If lung energy is too weak, pores do not close in time, allowing pathogens to penetrate and cause disorders. Lung *qi* vacuity can result in lowered resistance, which in turn can lead to increased susceptibility to colds. While the lungs are responsible for the control and distribution of defense *qi*, the center burner also contributes to the production of defense *qi*, along with the stomach and spleen. If those two organs are in a state of vacuity, *qi* supply of the whole body is lowered, which then affects quantity and quality of defense *qi*. Original essence (prenatal) *qi* from the kidneys also plays a minor role in the production of defense *qi*.

In summary, there are three energy systems responsible for good defense:

First and foremost, lung *qi* for governing and distributing defense *qi*, stomach and spleen *qi*, as well as for reproduction, quantity, and quality of defense *qi*. Secondly, original *qi* from the essence of liver *yang*. Thirdly, defense *qi* is a fleeting and active *yang* energy. With its role in the opening and closing of pores, it is closely associated with the secretion of body fluids (sweat). During the day, it circulates mostly in the surface *yang* channels of greater *yang* (*tai yang*) lesser *yang* (*shao yang*), and *yang ming*. At nighttime, it flows back into the bowels (*zang* organs) kidney, heart, lung, liver, and spleen.

Symptoms

General symptoms of *qi* or *yang* vacuity include: pale complexion; feeling cold, shivering and aversion to cold; cool and cold extremities; easily physically and emotionally fatigued; general listlessness; spontaneous perspiration (lung *qi* vacuity). During the acute phase of a cold: chills, a feeling of coldness along one's back along the greater *yang* (*tai yang*) channel, joint pain; runny nose with liquid, clear secretion; sneezing, sensitive to cold, exhaustion (symptoms of a wind-cold attack on the body).

Causes

- Factors that weaken lung *qi*, for example constitutional weakness, extended periods of sitting in a slumped position (inhibits breathing and thus leads to lung *qi* vacuity). Smoking, damage to lung *qi* by external pathogenic factors such as wind-cold or wind-heat, overwork, prolonged grief.
- Factors that weaken spleen and stomach.
- Factors that weaken kidney *yang* and essence.

Therapy

Strengthen body *yang*
激 • KI-7 + Moxa • ST-36 • GV-4

Supplement lung *qi*
激 • LU-9 + Moxa • LU-7
• BL-13 • BL-12

Supplement center burner
激 • ST-36 • BL-20

Supplement kidney *yang*
激 • KI-7 + Moxa • BL-23 • GV-4

Nutritional Therapy

Avoid:

All foods that can weaken the *yang* of the body, for example foods with cool or cold thermal nature such as raw foods, salads, cold types of fruit, dairy products, cold beverages.

During the **acute phase** of a common cold, avoid all foods that increase the formation of mucus to protect the weakened lung *qi* from possible phlegm disorders and to avoid straining the spleen (bananas, dairy products, raw foods, and very oily and fatty foods).

Recommended:

Acrid–warm and acrid–hot flavors that strengthen the metal phase to supplement and support defense *qi*.
During the acute beginning of a cold, avoid the sour flavor. In Chinese medicine, all citrus fruits are contraindicated for the duration of a cold. The reason is the direction of movement of the sour flavor. It moves inward and thus prevents the already weakened defense *qi* from coming to the surface and averting the penetrating pathogenic factors. This results in the pores of the skin being insufficiently closed, creating a relatively unobstructed path for entry of pathogenic factors through the skin. The sour flavor makes it possible for pathogenic factors located on the body surface to move into deeper layers. Thus, TCM believes hot lemon juice and large servings of citrus fruits such as oranges and lemons should not be consumed for the duration of a cold.

In Chinese herbal therapy, *huang qi* (astragalus) is an important remedy for supplementing defense *qi*.

In the early stage of a cold, it is especially productive to treat the symptoms (cold and chills) with the strong *yang* energy of acrid–warm and acrid–hot flavors. This moves defense *qi*, opens the pores for a short time to allow the expulsion of pathogenic factors such as cold, dispels external pathogenic cold and wind, clears the body surface, and strengthens *yang* and defense *qi* in the body.

Recommended:

Spices	Especially fresh ginger! Also pepper, chili, acrid spiced tea (e.g., yogi tea)

Decoction of fresh ginger with green (spring) onions:
Simmer thumb-sized pieces of fresh ginger and green onions in 0.5 L (two cups) of water for about 10 minutes. Drink one to two cups of this liquid while warm.

All foods with *yang* potential are recommended for strengthening defense *qi*. Sweet–warm or sweet–hot flavors are especially suitable for supplementing the center burner. Salty–hot and salty–warm flavors can strengthen the kidneys. The body is especially susceptible to pathogenic energy at night, since defense *qi* circulates deeper in the body during that time, leaving the surface unprotected. Too little sleep and too much nightly activity increase susceptibility to externally caused disorders.
Nutritional therapy can individually strengthen specific organs with certain foods. Aside from generally supplementing *yang* in the body via the three networks kidney, spleen/stomach, and lung, supplementing lung *qi* is especially advisable for strengthening the body's defenses.

Supplementing Lung *Qi*

Nutritional Therapy

Spices	Chili, curry, ginger, pepper
Beverages	Spiced teas, high-proof alcohol
Vegetables	Cauliflower, leeks, horseradish, onions, radish, watercress
Nuts and seeds	Almonds, almond butter

Wind-cold disorder, which attacks the lung when there is insufficient defense *qi* to protect it, can develop into wind-heat, which is characterized by fever; thirst, a preference for cold beverages, headaches, sparse, dark urine, and physical exhaustion. These signs of a wind-heat attack with predominant heat symptoms require immediate adjustment of nutritional therapy. During this phase, acrid-hot and acrid-warm flavors, as well as foods with a hot thermal nature are contraindicated; cooling foods are recommended. Sour flavors should be avoided to prevent the disorders from moving into deeper layers of the body.

Dampness and Phlegm Conditions

TCM views dampness and phlegm as important and common pathological factors in the treatment of many disorders.

The motto of traditional Chinese physicians was: "If you've treated a disorder for a long period of time without success, always remember phlegm."

The Western observer associates phlegm disorders mainly with a stuffed up nose and sinuses, sinusitis frontalis, sinusitis maxillaris, and bronchial congestion. In TCM, these are only partial aspects, as the Chinese idea of phlegm disorders incorporates a lot more than just material phlegm: Phlegm can occur in all parts of the body. It slows down the flow of *qi* and congests the channels, inducing symptoms such as numbness, dull, "foggy" headache, sluggishness, and lack of concentration.
A well-known and typical symptom of dampness in the head is the so-called hangover headache caused by too much alcohol resulting in the creation of phlegm.

Pathogenesis

Phlegm is created mainly by a disorder of the spleen/pancreas network. If the spleen is too weak, *qi* flow slows and transformation and transport of fluids becomes congested. As a result, dampness accumulates. With chronic spleen *qi* or *yang* vacuity, dampness collects over a longer period and creates concentrated accumulations of liquid. These eventually thicken into phlegm, especially if subjected to the effects of heat. Since spleen vacuity is always the primary cause of phlegm, therapy needs to focus on strengthening this particular bowel (*zang* organ)!
Also contributing to the formation of phlegm are the lungs and kidneys. The primary responsibility of the lungs is to distribute and reduce fluids produced by the spleen. If weakened, the lungs are unable to perform this task, resulting in the formation of dampness (swelling and edemas) and phlegm in the nasal and sinus cavities (maxillary sinus and frontal sinus). In the worst case, the lungs themselves become obstructed (bronchitis, pneumonia).
The kidneys, on the other hand, are responsible for the intake and discharge of liquids. If this function is impaired, liquids gather primarily in the lower burner and can lead to formation of edemas. As a rule, good kidney energy (kidney *yang*) is important for warming and supporting the spleen.
Other causes for the formation of phlegm, especially heat phlegm (viscous, yellow phlegm) are external wind-heat disorders that damage the lung, for example acute bronchitis, sinusitis, and hay fever. Heat phlegm can also arise with liver *qi* stagnation, since heat is formed when the flow of *qi* is slowed and congested, and heat thickens fluids.

Phlegm Differentiation

- *Substantial phlegm*: Appears in the form of sputum with disorders of the respiratory system, for example rhinitis, sinusitis, bronchitis, or pneumonia.
- *Immaterial, "invisible" phlegm*: Collects in the channels of the body and obstructs *qi* flow. Immaterial phlegm can gather subcutaneously and appear in the shape of skin nodules: Lipoma, adenoma, ganglia, or as a goiter. In its hardened form, phlegm turns into gallstones or

kidney stones. Phlegm in the joints causes bone deformation or chronic rheumatoid arthritis. Even "plum pit *qi*" (the sensation of a foreign body in the throat, *mei he qi*), a condition known in TCM, is another form of phlegm (*qi* phlegm), triggered mainly by binding depression of liver *qi* due to emotional causes. Its symptoms can include difficulty swallowing, globus hystericus ("lump in the throat"), or a feeling of oppression in the chest and diaphragm.

Symptoms

General phlegm disorders

- Protracted illnesses that do not improve despite intensive treatment.
- Painless lumps beneath the skin that are neither hot nor red and are freely movable (lipoma).
- A general feeling of heaviness and numbness, sluggishness, chronic fatigue, difficulty concentrating, especially dull headache and recurrent dizziness (Ménière disease).
- Frequent infections in children, with stuffy nose, muciferous and purulent bronchitis, and purulent maxillary sinus and frontal sinus infections.
- Obesity.

Tip: These symptoms can be increasingly found in children and young adults due to bad dietary habits (fast food, too many sweets, dairy products, and sugary soda pops).

Differentiation of phlegm disorders by location of phlegm collection and symptoms

- *Upper burner*: Fatigue, lack of concentration, dull pressure in head, dizziness, ringing in the ears (tinnitus), sinusitis frontalis and sinusitis maxillaris, stuffy nose.
- *Center burner*: Bronchitis, pneumonia, broncièctasis (inflammation of the lungs), cough with copious white or yellow secretion, nausea.
- *Lower burner*: Fluid deposits in the form of leg or ankle edemas.

Differentiation by type of phlegm condition and symptoms

- *Wind and phlegm*: Feeling of dizziness, sensation of numbness in the extremities, aphasia (communication disorder), wind stroke.
- *Heat phlegm*: Yellow, viscous sputum, dry mouth and lips, bronchitis, pneumonia, apathy, nebulous, confused mind, types of schizophrenia, hallucinations, manic depression.
- *Cold phlegm*: White, viscous sputum; lack of appetite, feeling of oppression in chest and epigastrium (abdominal wall above umbilicus [belly button]), infection of lungs.
- *Immaterial phlegm*: Congestion of the channels, for example wind colic (apoplexy) and sensation of numbness, mostly in elderly people.

Tongue: Puffy, wet tongue is typical, partly with impression (spleen *qi* or spleen *yang* vacuity). Often oily, soft fur appears on a normal, but pale tongue in the retrolingual region. *White fur*: cold phlegm; *yellow fur*: heat phlegm.

Pulse: Typical slippery pulse, similar to pulse of a pregnant woman.

Therapy

Strengthen spleen

Transform dampness and phlegm

Strengthen lung and kidneys

激 • ST-40 • CV-12 • PC-6 • ST-36 • SP-3 • BL-20 • BL-21

For chronic disorders

激 • KI-3 • KI-7 • BL-23 • LU-9 • BL-13

Nutritional Therapy

Avoid:

Foods that produce copious phlegm, especially dairy products, bananas, very oily and fatty foods, junk foods, too much of the sweet flavors, sugary beverages. An excess of *yin* foods (take into account season and climate!): raw foods, salads, and cool/cold types of fruit, citrus fruits, and juices. Frozen foods and cooking or heating meals in the microwave should also be avoided.

Caution: Meat and alcohol produce phlegm if consumed excessively. This applies especially to pork and wheat beer.

Recommended: Strengthen spleen

- All foods that strengthen the spleen to deter further production of dampness and phlegm (see "Spleen/Pancreas *Qi* Vacuity," p. 69 and "Spleen/Pancreas *Yang* Vacuity," p. 69).
- Millet, rice, and corn are especially beneficial for supplementing and warming the spleen.
- Soy beans and mung beans are recommended for removing excess moisture from the body.

Flavors and foods that transform dampness and phlegm:

- **Heat phlegm (yellow, viscous):**
- *Thermal nature/flavor:* bitter–cool, salty–cool, sometimes sweet–cool
- Belgian endive hearts, dandelion, soy milk, mung beans, radish, pears, grapes, carp, salt, red marine algae (rhodophyta, also known as dulse), and seaweed.
- ***Cold phlegm (whitish, clear, thin):***
  Thermal nature/flavor: bitter–warm, acrid–warm
  In moderation, fresh ginger, leeks, garlic, cardamom, cherries.
- Phlegm obstructs qi flow in the meridians:
- Moderately acrid flavor can remove the congestions, for example strong spices such as pepper, garlic, ginger.

> **Tip:** **With recurrent phlegm conditions, drastically reduce meat, alcohol, dairy products, sweets, and fatty foods. Abstain from these altogether for three to six weeks.**

General recommendation for dampness and phlegm: Millet muesli or millet porridge with cinnamon and raisins.
For heat phlegm: Mung beans, mung bean decoction, soy milk, mixed juice of pears and lemons.
For cold phlegm: Ginger tea.

B Application of Chinese Dietetics for Specific Conditions

Network:
• Spleen/Pancreas–Stomach
• Earth Phase

Bowel (*Zang* Organ): Spleen/Pancreas (*Pi*), SP

Character

"In charge of economy and nutrition"

The spleen is the material foundation of the body and root of acquired *qi*. It is responsible for absorption, distribution, transformation, and creation of energy from food.

Role in TCM:

- Governs transformation, transport, and processing of food and energy.
- Retains the blood in the blood vessels.
- Governs muscles and extremities.
- Opens at mouth and lips.
- Governs upbearing *qi*, keeps the organs in place.
- Houses the mind (*zhi*).

Association with the five phases:

- *Emotions*: Brooding, worries, pensiveness
- Climate factor: Dampness
- *Season*: Late summer, early fall
- *Direction*: Center
- *Color*: Yellow
- *Flavor*: Sweet
- Time of day: 9–11 a.m.

Viscera (*Fu* Organ): Stomach (*Wei*) ST

Function

"Cooking vessel" for acquired *qi*

- Most important viscera (*Fu* organ): Downbears the flow of *qi*
- Gathers food
- Separates and extracts food
- Downbears
- Loves dampness
- Time of day: 7–9 a.m.

Tasks and Functions of Spleen/Pancreas and Stomach

The stomach and spleen/pancreas are important bowels and viscera (*zang fu* organs). As the production site of acquired *qi*, *yang*, blood (*xue*), and body fluids (*jin ye*), they play a key role in TCM therapy. The famous Chinese scholar *Li Gao*, during the *Song* dynasty (AD 920–1280), emphasized the importance of the center burner by founding a special school for the "Strengthening of the Center," which focused primarily on the treatment of the center burner.

The following quote from the *Ming* Dynasty (AD 1368–1644) also speaks to the significance of the body's "center":

"The person who knows how to treat the center knows how to balance all networks."

Many doctors during that period were of the opinion that no disorder is really curable as long as the network of the center burner is impaired. They perfected strengthening the "inner center" by strengthening the stomach and spleen as a prerequisite for all therapy.

"*Zang Fu* Governs Transformation and Transport"

The bowels and viscera (*zang fu* organs) spleen/pancreas are largely responsible for transformation and transport of ingested food. Both organs separate food into clear and turbid components. The clear components of food essence are transformed into *gu qi* (drum *qi*). *Gu qi* forms the basis for all acquired *qi* and for production of blood. According to TCM, most of the *qi* in our body that can be regenerated is derived from *gu qi* acquired through stomach and spleen/pancreas. Lack of spleen *qi* results in energy deficiencies for the entire body.

Key symptoms of spleen *qi* vacuity:
Chronic fatigue, general immune deficiency, susceptibility to infections, lack of concentration; sloppy, shapeless stool.

Therapy

Therapy principle:
Supplementing *qi* means also supplementing the spleen. Strengthening blood means also supplementing the spleen.

Governance of Body Fluids and Liquids

Transformation and distribution of fluids requires sufficient spleen *qi*. Spleen vacuity obstructs the transport of fluids. This can cause accumulation of dampness or phlegm, which can damage a weakened spleen even further. The spleen loves dryness and shuns dampness. Dampness in the body can be caused by external wetness and dampness (damp apartment, rainy fall days), but also by dampness formed on the inside of the body caused by the wrong foods (too many *yin* foods).

Key factors that can weaken the spleen and cause dampness and later formation of phlegm, are excessive consumption of cold beverages, raw foods, salads, fruit and dairy products. Dampness, phlegm, or edemas in the body always requires treating the spleen as part of the therapy.

Symptoms

Edemas, swollen face, sensation of heaviness in the limbs; heavy, dull head; apathy, depression and lack of drive, obesity, sinus congestion (maxillary and frontal sinuses), bronchial congestion, frequent colds (see also "Dampness and Phlegm Conditions," p. 64)

Signs of healthy spleen *qi* include well-shaped red lips, a closed mouth, and a good sense of taste. Spleen *qi* vacuity presents as pale and chapped lips and a continually open mouth. A strong preference for sweet flavors also indicates spleen disharmony.

Production and Retention of Blood

Healthy spleen *qi* produces sufficient blood and enables it to circulate through the body and stay in its vessels. Spleen *qi* vacuity can cause more frequent bleeding, because the blood can not be retained in its vessels. *Gu qi* (drum *qi*) is extracted from food and then transported by the spleen to the heart. Blood is produced in the heart with help from the original *qi* of the kidneys. This makes the spleen one of the central organs for the formation of *qi* and blood. Chronic spleen *qi* vacuity reduces the production of blood and results in liver blood vacuity.

Symptoms

Night blindness; blurry, distorted vision; light-sensitive eyes; numb limbs; insomnia (*shen* is anchored in the blood), menstrual disorders, frequent bruises (purpura, petechia, hematuria, excessive menstruation).

Governance of Muscles and Limbs

Gu qi extracted by the spleen from food is distributed to all tissues of the body. This nourishes and warms muscles and limbs and supports mobility. Weak, tired, or atrophied muscles indicate spleen *qi* vacuity.

Governance of Connective Tissue

The spleen holds the organs in place. Taught and elastic connective tissue is a sign of good spleen *qi*. Loose connective tissue, cellulite, colon/rectal prolapse (*tuo gang*), or uterus prolapse (*zi gong xia chui*) indicate weak spleen *qi*.

Home of the Mind/Thought (*Si*)

Clear thinking and good concentration indicate strong spleen *qi*. Spleen vacuity can present as mental symptoms such as fuzzy thinking, problems concentrating, and weak memory

Tip: Mental overexertion can weaken the spleen, which explains a craving for sweets during long periods of intensive studying or other mental work. The sweet flavor is associated with the earth phase and, therefore, with the spleen. Sweet flavor has the strongest supplementing effect of all flavors. In moderation, eating sweet foods during times of intense mental activity (studying, writing) can be beneficial.

Honey, dates, poppy seed cake or muffins, raisins.

Special Diet for Spleen/ Pancreas–Stomach Network

This network is one of the most important sources of acquired *qi* and responds very well to dietary supplementation and treatment. The mainstay of every meal should be the sweet flavor of the earth phase. All other flavors should only be used as supplements (see also "Strengthening the Inner Center," p. 42).

- Sweet foods such as grains, poultry, vegetables, certain types of fruit and dried fruit strengthen *qi* and moisten body fluids; they strengthen and supplement our "center."
- Excessive consumption of cold beverages, raw foods, fruit, and dairy products weaken the spleen.
- Spleen *qi* vacuity caused by extended periods of mental activity and mental strain should be compensated with appropriate foods of the sweet flavor.
- ***Caution***: Excessive consumption of refined sugar and denatured sweeteners (so-called simple sugars) causes extreme fluctuations of blood glucose levels and depletes nutrients from the body. Concentrated "healthy" sweeteners such as honey, maple syrup, molasses, or raw cane sugar are also extreme representatives of the sweet flavor and should be consumed in moderation.
- Spleen vacuity causes dampness and phlegm. If present, dietary measures to treat the spleen should be included in treatment.

Spleen Syndromes and Chinese Nutrition

Spleen *qi* vacuity (*pi qi xu*)
Spleen *yang* vacuity (*pi yang xu*)

■ Spleen *Qi* Vacuity (*Pi Qi Xu*)

This is probably one of the most common syndromes found in clinical practice and leads patients into the doctor's office with a variety of different symptoms.

Western diagnosis:
Gastroenteritis, indigestion, malabsorption syndrome, diarrhea, anemia, and inflammatory intestinal disorders.

Symptoms
Chronic fatigue, general exhaustion, susceptibility to infection, lack of appetite, weakness and frailty of limbs, craving sweets; pale, pallid complexion; soft, sloppy stools; sometimes diarrhea.

■ Spleen *Yang* Vacuity (*Pi Yang Xu*)

Spleen *yang* vacuity can result from protracted spleen *qi* vacuity or pronounced weakening of the spleen due to cold foods, irregular meal times, and irregular eating habits.

Western diagnosis:
Chronic gastroenteritis, anemia, chronic malabsorption, and chronic gastroenterological disorders.

Symptoms

Feet and hands are always cold; shivering; a sensation of cold in the abdomen; watery stool with undigested food particles; edemas, weakness, fatigue, chronic digestive problems.

Pathogenesis

Four factors can weaken the spleen:

- Diet
- Mental strain
- Climate
- Chronic illness

Diet: Probably the number one factor leading to a weakening of spleen *qi*. Bad eating habits such as irregular meals, eating too late in the day (e.g., having the first warm meal of the day in the evening), overeating, excessive consumption of cold and raw foods (too many *yin* products), too much dairy, too much frozen food, heating and cooking foods in the microwave, excessive consumption of acrid spices, and too many *yin* foods during the cold season all contribute to a weakening of spleen *qi*.

Mental strain: Excessive mental activity and mental strain produce spleen *qi* vacuity. This syndrome is compounded by food eaten too hastily due to mental strain combined with time pressure and stress.

Climate: Since the spleen despises wetness and dampness, it is sensitive to all dampness, especially from protracted exposure to wet weather or damp living environments, which weaken the spleen.

Chronic illnesses: Protracted illness progressively weakens and exhausts the spleen and eventually also weakens the kidney organ network.

Therapy

Supplement spleen ***qi***

激 • SP-3 • SP-2 • BL-20 • BL-21 • ST-36 • CV-12 • Moxa

Avoid:
Cold or cooling *yin* foods; excess acrid flavors; excessive consumption of sweets, especially refined sugar. The most common ones are outlined below:

Fruits	Pineapples, oranges, bananas, kiwis, watermelons, lemons
Vegetables	Cucumbers, raw foods, excessive consumption of salads (especially during the cold season), tomatoes
Beverages	Cold or iced drinks; too much mineral water; energetically cool fruit juices (e.g., orange juice); black tea, green tea, wheat beer, light beer
Dairy products	Cottage cheese, farmer's cheese, cream cheese, milk, sour milk products (e.g., yogurt, kefir)

Recommended:
Regular meals; at least one warm meal a day. Sweet and warming foods such as:

Flavor	Sweet–hot, sweet–warm, sweet–neutral
Cooking method	Neutral and warming
Meat	Poultry, poultry broth, lamb, beef, beef stock, venison
Fish	Trout, salmon, tuna, shellfish
Fruit	Sweet apples, apricots, dates, jujube (Chinese dates), figs, sweet cherries, peaches, plums, raisins, red grapes
Vegetables	Fennel, cabbage, pumpkins, carrots, sweet potatoes, onions gently sautéed until transparent
Beverages	Fennel tea, spiced tea with cinnamon (yogi tea), mead, liqueurs, corn silk tea, licorice tea, red grape juice
Grains	Amaranth, oats, millet, polenta, short-grain (glutinous) rice, rice
Nuts and seeds	Peanuts, hazelnuts, pistachios, sesame, walnuts
Sweeteners	Maple syrup, barley malt, raw honey, marzipan, raisins, raw cane sugar (e.g., Rapadura), molasses
Spices	Aniseed, star anise, cayenne, pepper, fennel, ginger, cardamom, nutmeg, vanilla, cinnamon; also spices of the fire phase such as coriander, oregano, rosemary, thyme

Comment: Spleen syndromes are a domain of Chinese dietetics. Treatment duration is two to three months; eat regularly.

Millet porridge with raisins, cinnamon, nuts, and warming fruits for breakfast.

Organ Network Spleen/ Pancreas–**Stomach**

"Sea of food and liquids"

TCM views the stomach network as a very significant viscera (*fu* organ). Its tasks and functions are closely related to those of the spleen. The most important function of the stomach is the absorption of food and its distribution via the spleen. A person's overall state of health is very dependent on the constitution of the stomach. Traditional Chinese doctors often measured the prognosis and course of a disorder by looking at the energy condition of the stomach. A stomach supplied with sufficient *qi* promised a brief disorder and rapid recovery. If the stomach energy was weakened, the prognosis was unfavorable, since the formation of *qi* as well as the beneficial effect of herbs and acupuncture require a healthy stomach.

The task of the stomach is to separate and digest food. TCM believes that the stomach separates food into clear and turbid components. Pure, clear components are transported to the spleen. Impure, turbid components are eliminated via the intestines. Clear *gu qi* (drum *qi*) is distributed with the help of spleen and lungs. The stomach is seen as the origin of the acquired body fluids (*jin ye*) and thus of acquired *yin*, which is formed in the body with the help of kidney *yin*.

Dryness and heat are especially damaging to the stomach. Examples are foods with too much *yang* quality, such as acrid spices, coffee, high-proof alcohol or warming cooking methods, such as grilled or rapidly seared foods. Strong emotions such as anger, frustration, and resentment can also produce heat and attack the stomach. A healthy stomach requires a proper diet. The following recommendations should be considered: high food quality; regular meals (three to five meals a day); a substantial, leisurely breakfast; at least one warm meal a day. Do not eat too much or too little, do not eat too late in the evening, and do not eat when under time pressure (no "wolfing down" of meals). Chew well, between 10 and 15 times per bite.

Stomach problems may be closely related to spleen disharmony and have to be treated concurrently.

General Causes of Stomach Dysfunction

The main causes of stomach dysfunction include external pathogenic cold, heat, dryness; excess of energetically too hot or too cold foods; and irregular eating habits. While the spleen assures that clear *gu qi* (drum *qi*) reaches the upper burner, the stomach's task is to transport the turbid components downward into the intestines. Impairment of this function can lead to vomiting, which TCM calls "*qi* vomiting" (*qi ou*). The stomach is unable to downbear *qi*, and as a result, it counterflows pathologically upward.

Example

A good example for excess "external pathogenic cold" is what often happens to children who spend their summer eating ice cream, drinking cold sodas, and staying in a cold swimming pool for longer periods, or running around in wet swimsuits. This can cool down and block the sensitive stomach *qi* of children in particular, resulting in stomach pain and lack of appetite. If this cold penetrates the body more deeply, it can cause stomach *yang* vacuity with symptoms like nausea, vomiting, and diarrhea.

> *Tip:* Ginger or spiced tea, fennel tea

Acupuncture or, for children, acupressure; moxa if applicable.

> **Strengthen stomach *qi* and spleen *qi***
> 激 • PC-6! • ST-36 • CV-12

- **Unfavorable eating habits**

Avoid eating too quickly and hastily, skipping breakfast, or insufficient breakfast. The best time for building up stomach *qi* is in the morning between 7 and 9 a.m.

Avoid irregular mealtimes, discussions at mealtime, and business lunches or dinners with exhausting conversations.

Avoid eating too late in the evening or during the night (weak period for the stomach).

If the stomach is filled with too much food during its weak period, it is unable to transform and transport the food. This results in "food stagnation" in the stomach, accompanied by bloating and disturbed sleep. Protracted weakening of stomach *qi* weakens stomach *yin*. Obesity is a common consequence of this condition.

Frequently changing diets, following unbalanced nutritional advice, and fasting lead first to stomach *qi* vacuity, then to spleen *qi* vacuity, and may reduce the overall *qi* and *yang* of the body. During times of stress, it is especially important to concentrate on a balanced and regular diet.

- **Emotional factors**

Emotional stress factors, especially anger and worry, have a distinct adverse impact on stomach function. A Chinese saying advises not eating immediately after an argument, so that the *qi* has time to calm down first. Sudden food cravings and eating out of frustration can be symptoms of unbalanced stomach *qi*. Strong (or suppressed) emotions can give rise to depressed *qi*, which then transforms into fire (Wiseman) and can cause sudden cravings. *Qi* stagnation caused by suppressed or intense emotions can also block the flow of *qi* in stomach, spleen, and even lungs. The resulting food stagnation prevents food from being trans-

Foods that weaken stomach function	
Cold foods Raw foods, salad, ice cream, fruit, cold drinks	Cool stomach and spleen
Hot foods Acrid spices such as pepper, curry, garlic, or ginger	Damage stomach, create stomach heat
Yang foods Lamb, alcoholic beverages	Damage stomach, create stomach heat
Sugar and sweets	Create dampness and phlegm, which weaken the spleen and damage stomach due to heat
Fatty foods	Create dampness and phlegm

formed properly. As a result, the body is not supplied with sufficient *qi*. Frequently, food passes through the digestive tract and is eliminated only partially digested (*wan gu bu hua*, or nontransformation of food), and little use is made of the potential food energy (spleen vacuity with food damage, or *pi xu jia shi*). As a result, stomach and *qi* are not supplied with sufficient acquired *qi* and weakened in case of protracted emotional obstruction. Other factors involving the stomach are physical and mental exhaustion, congenital weakness, and even the wrong treatment strategies or medicines.

Stomach Syndromes and Chinese Nutrition

Stomach *qi* vacuity (*wei qi xu*)
Stomach *yin* vacuity (*wei yin xu*)
Stomach *qi* vacuity with cold (*wei qi xu han*)
Food stagnation in the stomach (*shi zhi wei wan [guang]*)
Stomach heat (*wei re*)

Stomach *Qi* Vacuity (*Wei Qi Xu*)

This syndrome is very similar to spleen *qi* vacuity. The prime time of activity for the stomach is in the morning between 7 and 9 a.m. A major share of our food for the day should be eaten during that time to enable us to produce the energy needed for the day. If stomach *qi* is vacuous, spleen *qi* is depleted as well, resulting in symptoms like lack of appetite, fatigue, and general weakness.

Western diagnosis:
Lack of appetite, diarrhea, nausea, lack of appetite in children, weakness during recovery, rectal prolapse (tuo gang).

Symptoms

Morning fatigue, lack of appetite (especially in children), upper abdominal complaints, and sloppy stool.

Tongue: Pale, floppy, sometimes enlarged
Pulse: Vacuous

Causes

Diet: The most common cause of stomach *qi* vacuity is insufficient and inappropriate diet: Eating irregularly, eating too much or too little, fatty food; one-sided, unbalanced diets.
General: Chronic illnesses

Therapy

Supplement stomach *qi* and spleen *qi*
激 • ST-36 • CV-12 • BL-21
• SP-2 • BL-20 • Moxa

Recommended:

Thermal Nature	Warm, neutral
Flavor	Sweet–warm, sweet–neutral
Cooking Method	Warming

See also "Spleen *Qi* Vacuity," page 69 and "Spleen *Yang* Vacuity," page 69.

Stomach *qi* vacuity is always treated the same as spleen *qi* or spleen *yang* vacuity in nutritional therapy. Dietary measures should keep the stomach sufficiently damp. This might require incorporating more neutral or gently cooling foods into the diet. Since the stomach, unlike the spleen, loves dampness and hates dryness, fewer hot and dry foods should be used for stomach *qi* vacuity than for spleen *yang* vacuity. Besides dietary measures, good eating habits and proper diet are important steps toward long-term stabilization of the stomach.

Comment/Prognosis

A well-functioning stomach and a "strong" spleen are key ingredients in the overall formation and preservation of *qi* in the body. Developing good eating habits is as important as choosing the right foods. Both should be maintained long term. Within days or weeks, the patient will feel a noticeable difference. Dietary measures are simple ways to permanently correct dysfunctions that have persisted for years, such as feelings of pressure in the epigastric region, nausea, and lack of appetite. Adopting a lifestyle that is supportive to spleen, stomach, and center burner is advisable for maintaining good energy, a strong immune system, and lasting vitality.

Stomach *Yin* Vacuity (*Wei Yin Xu*)

Stomach *yin* vacuity is a commonly found syndrome caused mostly by poor dietary habits, but also by chronic heat disorders of the stomach. Stomach *yin* vacuity frequently results from longstanding damaging factors.

Western diagnosis:
Chronic gastritis, gastric insufficiency, chronic nausea and vomiting, gastric and duodenal ulcers.

Symptoms

Lack of appetite, lethargy, afternoon fever or heat sensation, constipation (dry, hard stools), dry mouth, thirst without the desire to drink, drinking in small portions, bloating after eating, minimal to moderate pains in the solar plexus (epigastrium), bleeding gums.

Tongue: Red, dry, clean (without fur); no fur in center

Pulse: Thin, rapid

Causes

Diet: The main causes of stomach *yin* vacuity are unfavorable dietary and eating habits, such as late evening meals; rushed, hectic meals; starting work right after eating; chronic heat disorders of the stomach and chronic stomach *qi* vacuity.

General: Chronic illnesses, syndromes that expose spleen to protracted heat and dampness.

Aging leads to a physiological stomach *yin* vacuity.

Pathogenesis

The stomach loves dampness and is regarded as a source of *yin*. When the stomach is weakened, dryness forms in the body ("hot" foods, coffee, acrid spiced tea). A diagnostic indicator of stomach *yin* vacuity is a red tongue without tongue fur, especially in the center of the tongue, which represents the stomach area. This is caused by a lack of dampness. The stomach functions properly when it is heated by the lower burner. This vaporizes stomach liquids, which then rise into the upper burner and settle on the tongue as a whitish coating (fog). These physiological signs of a healthy stomach are missing with *yin* vacuity, since no fluids are available to be vaporized.

Therapy

Nourish stomach *yin*

激 • SP-3 • SP-6 • KI-3

Replenish body fluids

激 • ST-36 • CV-12

Avoid:

Thermal nature	Warm, hot foods
Flavor	Bitter–hot, bitter–warm, acrid–hot, acrid–warm
Beverages	High-proof alcohol, coffee, red wine, black tea
Spices	Acrid spices
Other	Grilled, broiled, or barbecued foods

Recommended:

Thermal nature	Mostly neutral and cooling foods that have a refreshing effect and replenish fluids; possibly slightly warming foods in moderation
Cooking method	Cooling, fluid-forming cooking methods
Flavor	Sweet–neutral, sweet–cool, sweet–cold
Meat	Poultry and beef in the form of soups or stews, pork, rabbit, goose
Fruit	Apples, pears, bananas, tangerines, honeydew melons
Vegetables	Cauliflower, napa (Chinese) cabbage cucumbers, watercress, raw foods, salads, celeriac (celery root), steamed tomatoes, zucchini, eggplant, potatoes

Beverages	Pear juice, bread drink (a lacto-fermented beverage made from grain), rosehip tea, corn silk tea, mallow tea (hibiscus palustris or swamp rose-mallow), milk, soy milk, red grape juice, wheat beer
Grains	Spelt, millet, rice, short-grain (glutinous) rice, wheat
Other	Milk products, butter, egg, cheese, cream

! In dietary therapy, vegetable casseroles baked in the oven are especially beneficial for replenishing body fluids in case of stomach syndromes.

Comment/Prognosis

Stomach *yin* vacuity calls first and foremost for a change in dietary habits and the right food choices. These two therapy approaches will produce significant improvement after just a few weeks or months. Patients will subjectively experience a distinct improvement of stomach disorders and a general increase in strength and vitality.

Appropriate lifestyle and diet can eliminate stomach disorders permanently. Restoring stomach function often resolves other disorders brought on by a deficiency of liquids and body fluids. Dietary therapy is especially well suited for alleviating symptoms in women with gynecological disorders rooted in blood vacuity. Elderly people often find a distinct improvement of long-lasting constipation problems.

■ Stomach *Qi* Vacuity with Cold (*Wei Qi Xu Han*)

This syndrome can appear in combination with spleen *yang* vacuity. Kidney *qi* can be impacted or damaged as well. This condition is generally caused by diets containing an excess of *yin* products.

Stomach *qi* vacuity with cold and spleen *yang* vacuity are closely connected. Symptoms include cold extremities, sloppy stools, and vomiting of clear fluids. Coldness and emptiness in the stomach can be improved by warm meals and beverages, but also by external application of heat and massages, since these supply the body with *yang*.

Western diagnosis:
Lack of appetite, recurrent nausea and vomiting, chronic diarrhea, uncomfortable feeling or sensation of coldness in the solar plexus (epigastrium).

Symptoms

Uncomfortable feeling of pressure in the solar plexus (epigastrium) that is generally improved by heat (hot-water bottle) or pressure. Discomfort often worsens after bowel movement. Symptoms improve with eating. Lack of appetite, dislike of cold beverages, preference for warm beverages and warm foods, vomiting of clear fluid, no thirst, sloppy stools, and cold extremities with a sensation of heaviness.

Causes

Diet: Cold foods; chronic excess of salads, raw foods, fruit, ice-cold beverages, ice cream, etc.

General: External pathogenic cold (wet swimsuit); can also be caused by invasive abdominal surgery.

Therapy

Warm stomach and spleen
激 • CV-12 • CV-6 • ST-36 • Moxa

Supplement kidney
激 • KI-3 • KI-7 • BL-23 • Moxa

Avoid:

Thermal nature	Cooling, especially cold foods
Cooking method	Cooling
Flavor	No special recommendations

Recommended:

Thermal nature	Warm, hot foods
Cooking method	Warming
Flavor	Sweet–hot, sweet–warm, bitter–warm, bitter–hot
Foods	All foods that strengthen the center burner (see "Spleen Qi Vacuity," p. 69 and "Spleen Yang Vacuity," p. 69)

Drink one cup of ginger tea every morning.

Comment/Prognosis

Consistent implementation of dietary recommendations can bring about distinct improvements with this syndrome within a few days or weeks. When combined with acupuncture or moxibustion, this syndrome can be easily treated. Continued adoption of dietary recommendations can stabilize the stomach in the long term.

Food Stagnating in the Stomach (*Shi Zhi Wei Wan*)

This syndrome often appears with excessive intake of food at the wrong time, especially big dinners and "holiday feasts."

Western diagnosis:
Indigestion, insomnia, abdominal distention (meteorism), nausea, headaches.

Symptoms

Stomach *qi* is obstructed in its downbearing function by food retention. This causes a pathological upbearing of stomach *qi* with the following symptoms: Bloating in the solar plexus (epigastrium) alleviated by vomiting; nausea, vomiting, burping, sour reflux, bad breath, lack of appetite.
Protracted stomach *qi* vacuity with cold can also obstruct heart *qi*. This leads to restlessness at night and disturbed sleep.

This repletion syndrome can appear in the form of cold or heat. To differentiate the two, look at tongue fur: white = cold, yellow = heat.

Causes

Diet: Common causes are overeating, hasty or hurried meals, and eating while under psychological or emotional strain.

Therapy

Remove food stagnation
激 • ST-36 • LR-3 • SP-4

Downbear (*jiang*) stomach *qi*
激 • CV-10 • PC-6 • CV-12

Healthy eating habits: Allowing enough time, chewing carefully, and eating an appropriate amount (not too much, not too little).

- Digestive liqueurs: Aniseed, caraway seeds, herbal liqueurs
- *Also*: Barley, carrots, coriander, fennel, ginger, millet, vinegar, white cabbage

Stomach Fire (*Wei Re*)

This repletion heat syndrome dries out body fluids, causing intense thirst, constipation, and a dry tongue. Subsequent "upbearing" heat in the stomach channel causes swollen and bleeding gums. The repletion condition also prevents stomach *qi* from downbearing, resulting in esophageal (sour) reflux. In extreme cases, stomach fire combined with phlegm can impair the spirit (*shen*). This can lead to disturbed sleep and psychological symptoms. Protracted exposure to extreme heat (fire) can damage stomach substance (*yin* damage, frustration).

Western diagnosis:
Gastritis, ventricular and duodenal ulcers, stomatitis, nosebleeds.

Symptoms

Burning and pain in solar plexus (epigastrium), thirst, craving cold beverages, excessive appetite, food cravings, bleeding gums, sour reflux, vomiting after eating, nausea, bad breath, constipation.

Tongue: Reddish, enlarged; yellow, sometimes dry tongue fur. *For heat phlegm*: Thick, yellow, sticky tongue fur.

Pulse: Replete, deep, rapid. *For heat phlegm*: Slippery, rapid, replete.

Causes

Diet: Excess hot foods and warming cooking methods, especially acrid spices or coffee; smoking. *For heat phlegm*: Too much hot and fatty food, for example deep-fried foods.

General: Too many heated emotions, anger, too much brooding.

Therapy

Cool and remove stomach heat

激 • ST-44 • ST-45 • CV-12

Downbear stomach *qi*

激 • PC-6 • CV-10 • CV-13

Avoid:

Thermal nature	Hot and warm foods
Cooking method	Warming
Flavor	Bitter–hot, bitter–warm, acrid–hot, acrid–warm, sweet–hot, sweet–warm
Meat	Lamb
Beverages	High-proof alcohol, coffee, red wine
Spices	Chili, curry, ginger, garlic, pepper
Other	Smoked, fatty foods, strongly seasoned foods

Recommended:

Thermal nature	Cool, cold foods
Flavor	Sweet–cold, sweet–cool, bitter–cold, bitter–cool, sour–cold, sour–cool
Cooking method	Cooling
For stomach fire:	
Fruit	Pears, rhubarb, watermelons, bananas, honeydew melons, kiwis
Vegetables	Cucumber, mung beans, sprouts, tomatoes, peas, spinach, bamboo sprouts, Chinese (napa) cabbage
Beverages	Chamomile tea, green tea, black tea, wheat beer
Dairy products	Yogurt
Other	Tofu, wheat, dandelion

Since chamomile tea is cooling, it is recommended only for stomach fire and is contraindicated for cold stomach syndromes.

For phlegm symptoms:
Avoid muciferous foods

Comment/Prognosis

This syndrome can be successfully treated in a few days or weeks by changing eating habits and making the right food choices. It responds very well to a combination of dietary measures and acupuncture. Treatment needs to address the emotional factors leading to stomach heat. Heated discussions, arguments, and relationship or work problems can be even more detrimental than the effects of coffee or other foods with yang characteristics. In TCM, emotional strain and burdens play a far bigger role than they do in Western medicine!

Organ Network:
• Lung–Large Intestine
• Metal Phase

Bowel (*Zang* Organ): Lung (*Fei*), LU

Character

"In charge of foreign affairs and defense"
Controls the body's surface, is in direct contact with the environment, and is responsible for immune defense and most secretions.

Role in TCM:

- Dominates *qi* and governs breathing
- Governs diffusion and downbearing
- Governs regulation of waterways
- Houses the corporeal soul (*po*)
- Governs tissues, including skin and sweat glands, pores, and body hair
- Opens at the nose

Association with the five phases:

- *Emotion*: Sadness
- Climate factor: Dryness
- *Season*: Fall
- Direction: West
- *Color*: White, silver
- *Flavor*: Acrid
- Time of day: 3–5 a.m.

Viscera (*Fu* Organ): Large Intestine (*Da Chang*)

Function

Governs transformation and conveyance of waste: receives the turbid and firm parts passed down from the small intestine and forms it into stool before discharging it from the body. Downbearing lung *qi* supports the large intestine in defecating.

Organ Network Lung–Large Intestine

Governs *qi* and breathing

One of the most important functions of the lungs is to inhale air and transform it into clear, ancestral (or gathering) *qi* (*zong qi*), which it then combines with *gu qi* (drum *qi* from food) from the spleen. These are then combined with the essential *qi* (*jing*) into true *qi* (*zheng qi*). True *qi* is circulated in the meridians by the lungs to fill the body and nourish the organs. The lungs, together with the spleen, carry a major responsibility for the acquired *qi* in the body. True *qi* divides into two separate forms: channel *qi* (*yin qi*) and defense *qi* (*wei qi*). Defense *qi* protects against external pathogenic attacks such as cold or heat and is produced mainly from lung *qi*. TCM believes that sufficient, freely coursing lung *qi* is the foundation of a good defense (immune system).

Governs regulation of waterways, diffusion, and downbearing

Another important lung function is diffusion and downbearing of *qi* and governance of body fluids. Conveyance disorders in *qi* distribution lead to cough, pressure, and a restricted feeling in the thorax. Body fluids are connected with stomach function. The stomach gathers fluids and the lung network diffuses them throughout the body to keep the body moistened.

Symptoms

Water retention, edemas, eyelid edemas, but also dryness.

Governs skin

Skin dryness and blemishes, often caused by internal heat, damp heat, and a deficiency of body fluids, are very receptive to nutritional therapy.

Nutrition and Organ Network

Nutritional therapy is well suited for prevention of lung disorders—by supplementing lung *qi*—and for treatment of acute and chronic lung network disorders.

- Supplementing lung *qi* for overall good *qi* supply.
- Strengthening defense *qi*.
- During the acute phase of colds, but also as adjunct therapy during chronic illnesses, for example asthma, in combination with other therapies, such as acupuncture and healing herbs.
- For dry skin and mucous membranes by making use of cool and moistening foods.
- For phlegm disorders of the respiratory system, such as bronchitis, sinusitis, by strengthening the lung and spleen networks. Especially important for chronic phlegm conditions to prevent continued production of phlegm, but also to transform phlegm.
- Sadness as an emotional factor for lung disorders can be treated in nutritional therapy with acrid flavors and their dispersing effect.

Lung Syndromes and Chinese Nutrition

Lung *qi* vacuity (*fei qi xu*)
Phlegm-damp obstructing the lung (*tan shi zu fei*)
Lung *yin* vacuity (*fei yin xu*)

■ Lung *Qi* Vacuity (*Fei Qi Xu*)

In Chinese medicine, the lungs are known as the "delicate" organ. The lungs are the only *yin* organ with an external orifice via the respiratory tract and a direct connection with bioclimatic factors.
The lungs' susceptibility to external bioclimatic factors like wind-cold and wind-heat depends on the strength of defense *qi*, which is governed and diffused by the lungs. Defense *qi* is a barrier against external bioclimatic factors, which cannot damage the lung network as long as defense *qi* is strong enough. Lung *qi* vacuity is a syndrome commonly seen in practice.

Symptoms

Shortness of breath, quiet voice, pale complexion, shivering, susceptibility to infections; recurring respiratory infections like colds, flu, tonsillitis, bronchitis, asthma, pneumonia; moderate exhaustion.

Causes

General: Lung *qi* vacuity can be caused by external bioclimatic factors, especially wind- cold and wind-heat, or by congenital constitutional weakness. Smoking is detrimental to lung *qi*, as is prolonged or unresolved grief. Sitting hunched over with tense shoulders for extended periods of time is just as detrimental to lung *qi*, because it blocks the flow of the lung's main pathway. Taking frequent breaks from sitting for stretching or regular *qi gong* exercises that stimulate lung *qi* flow are beneficial. Such exercises also invigorate a tired mind.

Diet: Too many cold or cool food items or *yin* products.

Therapy

Supplement lung *qi*
激 • LU-9 • BL-13 • BL-12 • CV-6

Stimulate *qi* diffusion
激 • LU-7

In the engendering cycle (*sheng* cycle), the lung is the child of the earth phases spleen and stomach. Treating lung disharmony, therefore, is facilitated by feeding the child through supplementation of spleen and stomach.

Recommended:

All foods that supplement the center burner; foods used for treatment of lung *qi* vacuity:

Flavor	Acrid–warm, possibly slightly acrid–hot, as well as sweet–warm for supplementing spleen and stomach
Fish	Tuna, carp
Meat	Duck, quail
Fruit	Peaches, grapes
Vegetables	Cauliflower, kohlrabi, carrots, olives, onions, mushrooms
Grains	Oats, millet, barley malt, rice (roast lightly before preparing)
Spices	Ginger, garlic, thyme
Nuts and seeds	Peanuts
Other	High-proof alcohol

Colds that frequently occur during the cold fall and winter months, such as flu and bronchitis, can be prevented by timely strengthening of lung *qi* with a warming diet focused on acrid–warm flavors and by supplementing the center burner. Combined with sufficient physical activity or exercise in fresh air, this treatment strategy can successfully prevent recurring colds and the use of antibiotics.

Ginger tea every morning; increase use of strong seasoning.

Phlegm–Damp Obstructing the Lung (*Tan Shi Zu Fei*)

This syndrome encompasses several lung phlegm syndromes:
Phlegm–damp obstructing the lung (*tan shi zu fei*), phlegm–heat coating the lung (*tan re zu fei*, and phlegm–liquid coating the lung (*tan shui zu fei*). In practice, phlegm, phlegm–cold or phlegm–heat coating the lung is often a cold that has turned into bronchitis. Factors promoting the production and accumulation of phlegm include defense *qi* and lung *qi* vacuity, as well as a weakened spleen that insufficiently transforms and transports fluids. These fluids accumulate, are transformed into phlegm, and in the sequence of the engendering cycle (*sheng* cycle), are handed from the "mother phase" earth/spleen to the "child phase" metal/lung. Energetic spleen vacuity impairs the lung network in the engendering cycle. The phlegm produced by the spleen is stored in the lungs. In TCM, all respiratory disorders involving phlegm— from acute purulent bronchitis, chronic bronchitis, to acute or chronic frontal or maxillary sinusitis—are part of the same syndrome category. Acute phlegm disorders are relatively easy to treat with nutritional therapy. When the recommended dietary measures are strictly and consistently followed, nutritional therapy can also successfully treat recurrent and chronic congestion of the respiratory tract. By comparison, acupuncture alone is often insufficient therapy for treating these conditions in practice.

Chinese pathophysiology differentiates between cold and warm phlegm syndromes.

Cold phlegm is easy to cough up, of a whitish, transparent color, usually of a thin consistency, and displays excess cold.
Hot phlegm (phlegm–heat or phlegm–fire) is more difficult to cough up, and depending on clinical and pathogenic factors, is viscous, yellowish, or greenish, possibly even blood-colored and can smell bad or even rotten. This condition clearly displays excess heat.
Each condition requires a different treatment strategy.

Cold phlegm calls for warming treatment, for example supplementing acupuncture and warming, *yang*-inducing foods or Chinese herbs.
Hot phlegm calls for cooling, calming treatment with acupuncture, cooling Chinese herbs, and cooling foods. When treating phlegm–heat conditions with cooling foods, make sure that the weak spleen *qi* or the lungs are not further weakened (see "Dampness and Phlegm Conditions," p. 64)

Cough with sputum, dyspnea, asthma, chest tightness, headaches.

Causes

Lung obstructions involve the factors leading to lung *qi* vacuity discussed earlier (see "Lung *Qi*

Vacuity," p. 79 and "Defense *Qi* Vacuity," p. 62), as well as factors that can weaken the spleen and stomach.

Therapy

Loosen phlegm

激 • ST-40 • LU-5 • CV-22

Strengthen spleen and lungs

激 • SP-3 • BL-20 • BL-21 • ST-36 • LU-9 • BL-13 • LU-7

Avoid:

Foods that promote the formation of fluids and phlegm, such as dairy products, fatty, overly sweet or acrid foods, alcohol, bananas, and junk food.

Recommended:

Foods that supplement spleen *qi* and lung *qi*.

Flavor	Sweet–neutral, sweet–warm (spleen qi), bitter–cool (drying), acrid–warm (lung qi)
Fruit	Pears, star fruit, tangerines
Vegetables	Radish, asparagus, water chestnuts, lotus root, dandelion, Chinese (napa) cabbage
Grains	Millet, rice, rye, buckwheat
Spices	Fresh ginger, marjoram, pepper, cardamom
Nuts and seeds	Apricot seeds, almonds, walnuts

Foods for treating phlegm–heat conditions

Vegetables	Watercress, white radish, celeriac (celery root)
Beverages	Peppermint tea, lemon
Spices	Less acrid
Other	Soy beans, red seaweed (dulse), grapefruit, tangerines

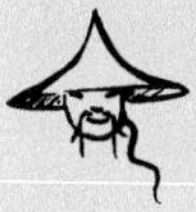

Lemon juice, green tea, pear juice.

Foods for treating cold phlegm conditions

Beverages	Bitter liqueurs (warm the body and remove dampness)
Spices	Garlic, ginger, pepper, cinnamon, thyme, cardamom
Other	Cherries, millet

Ginger tea

Foods for treating lung heat conditions

Fruit	Apples, pears
Vegetables	Savoy cabbage, asparagus, radish, carrots, dandelion, tomatoes, mushrooms
Other	Green tea, peppermint tea, mung beans, soy milk, salt, seaweed

Lung *Yin* Vacuity (*Fei Yin Xu*)

Prolonged exposure to external or internal heat attacks the body, dries up fluids, and damages lung *yin*. This syndrome can also result from chronic illness of other organs and long-term phlegm–heat syndrome.

Western diagnosis:
Chronic pharyngitis, bronchiectasis, chronic febrile bronchitis, chronic rhinitis, sinusitis, chronic cough, tuberculosis.

Symptoms

Dehydration of body fluids resulting in general dryness: Dry cough, dry mouth, and throat, hoarseness, sore throat, night sweat; subfebrile (below normal) body temperature, especially in the afternoon; sleep disturbances with hot flashes. Five hot areas on the feet, hands, and behind the sternum; hoarse voice; pale face with rosy cheeks; rosy cheeks in the afternoon or evening.

Tongue: Red, dry, chapped; little tongue fur. The more red and chapped the tongue, the more serious the condition.

Pulse: Rapid, floating pulse, in which the *yang* appears on the surface

Causes

General: Dryness; dehydration caused, for example by *yang* heat during hyperactivity; exhaustion of *yin*; smoking.

Diet: Too many warm–bitter foods, for example too much coffee; too many acrid–hot or acrid–warm foods that dry out body fluids; too much high-proof alcohol. Can also result from stomach *yin* vacuity, often caused by irregular meals, eating late in the evening, or hurried meals.

Elderly patients often suffer from lung *yin* vacuity due to insufficient body fluids.

Therapy

Enrich lung *yin*
激 • LU-9 • BL-13 • KI-6

Remove heat
激 • LU-5 • LU-6 • LU-10

Replenish body fluids
激 • KI-6 • CV-12 • SP-6

Avoid:
All warming foods and cooking methods that dry out body fluids even further and can produce heat in the body: acrid–hot, acrid–warm, bitter–hot, and bitter–warm flavors; foods with hot thermal nature.

Recommended:
Slightly cooling, neutral foods

Foods that moisten

Cooking method	Cooling
Flavor	Sweet, sweet–neutral, sweet–cool
Flavor	Banana (with honey), pear, tangerine, honeydew melon
Beverages	Poultry broth, almond milk, cow's milk
Nuts and seeds	Peanuts, almonds, sunflower seeds, sesame
Other	Marzipan, cottage cheese, farmer's cheese, butter, honey

Grandma's "milk with honey remedy" is still a suitable treatment for lung *yin* vacuity, especially for dry cough. Back in her days, tuberculosis—a lung *yin* vacuity syndrome—was common. However, this remedy is contraindicated for all phlegm conditions such as bronchitis, sinusitis, and colds, and is frequently used incorrectly.

Organ Network:
• Kidney–Bladder
• Water Phase

Bowel (*Zang* Organ): Kidney (*Shen*), KI

Character

"The Vice President"

"The lung is the governor of *qi* and the kidney is the root of *qi*" (Wiseman). The kidneys are the foundation of life, keeper of the original essence (*jing*), foundation of *yin* and *yang*, and seat of "fire and water" in the body.

Role in TCM:

- Kidney stores essence and governs birth, development, reproduction, and aging (*shen cang jing*)
- Kidney governs water (*shen zhu shui*)
- Kidney governs *qi* absorption (*shen zhu na qi*)
- Kidney stores mind/memory—governs willpower (*shen cang zhi*)

Association with the five phases

- *Emotion:* Fear
- Climate factor: Cold
- *Season:* Winter
- Direction: North
- *Color:* Blue, black
- Flavor: Salty
- *Time of day:* 5–7 p.m.

Viscera (*Fu* Organ): Bladder (*Pang Guang*)

Function

Receives the "turbid" fluids from small intestine and kidneys and stores and discharges them in the form of urine.

Keeps the lower waterways clear and open. The *Sue Wen* states in Elementary Questions: "The bladder holds the office of river island, stores fluid, and by (kidney) *qi* transformation, lets it out."

- Time of day: 3–5 p.m.

Organ Network Kidney–Bladder

- **"The kidney is the root of all *yang* and all *yin* in the body"**

This classic quote accurately describes the overall significance of the kidney network. Long-lasting imbalance and chronic illnesses weaken the kidney, which means it has to be strengthened as part of any therapy for chronic illness.

- **Kidney stores essence, governs birth, development, reproduction, and aging**

Kidney *yin* serves as a material basis for the development and maturation of egg cells and sperm. Kidney *yang* provides the energy for sexual activity. Kidney vacuity leads to a multitude of disorders such as impotence, weak libido, infertility, problems during pregnancy, and other sexual and urological dysfunctions.

Congenital *jing* (essence) is stored in the kidney organ network. This *jing* can be preserved, but not replenished. Acquired *jing*, which supplements congenital *jing*, is obtained through the daily intake of food.

- **Kidney governs water**

The kidney governs all production and movement of body fluids and via its connection with the bladder, is also responsible for the discharge of fluids. Excessive dryness, for example due to heat, weakens body fluids and kidney *yin*. The salty flavor associated with the kidney network is able to replenish fluids due to its hygroscopic properties.

- **Kidney rules *ming men*, the "fire of life" (*ming men zhi huo*)**

Cold—external cold (cold weather) as well as a diet that is energetically too cold—reduces and blocks kidney *yang* and causes lasting obstruction of all bodily functions. As the "fire of life" (*ming men zhi huo*), kidney *yang* warms the *yang* of the entire body. "*Ming men*," the life gate (GV-4), is also sometimes called the "gate of fire," the root of fire of all internal organs. The cold symptoms of chronic *yang* vacuity can be treated very effectively with nutritional therapy along with moxibustion, acupuncture, and Chinese herbs.

Nutrition and Organ Network

As a rule, only vacuity patterns develop in the kidney network. A good diet protects *jing* and kidney *qi*. For the kidney network, the focus should be on preventive dietary measures that support kidney *yang* and kidney *yin* long term to keep them from being exhausted.

Kidney *yang* is closely connected to both spleen *yang* and lung *qi*. Dietary measures should supplement **all three** networks: kidney, spleen, and lung.

Kidney Syndromes and Chinese Nutrition

Disharmony in the kidney network presents as vacuity or emptiness. The most important syndromes for nutritional therapy are:

Kidney *qi* vacuity (*shen qi xu*)
Kidney *yang* vacuity (*shen yang xu*)
Kidney *yin* vacuity (*shen yin xu*)

Kidney vacuity involves general physical weakness, as well as increased susceptibility to external and internal illnesses. Often appearing in connection with kidney vacuity are sexual dysfunction, urological conditions, and disorders of the lower back and bones.

Western diagnosis:
General weakness, sensitivity to cold, loss of strength, incontinence, enuresis (bedwetting), impotence, premature ejaculation, knee pain, chronic cystitis (urinary tract infections), nephritis, frigidity, depression, anxiety, chronic degenerative arthropathy, rheumatoid arthritis.

Pathogenesis

Regardless of the type of kidney disorder, the factors weakening kidney energy are similar. They differ only in severity and duration, which is determined by the gravity of the disorder and pathology of the network. *Qi* vacuity is a relatively mild disorder of the network. It can develop into a more serious disorder with *yang* vacuity symptoms if it persists and the damage increases. More severe damage can injure the organ system structure and present with the same symptoms as *yin* vacuity. Progression of disorders is not always so clear-cut and may involve gradual transitions and the involvement of other networks.

The most common cause weakening the energy exchange of the kidneys are the strong demands made on the body by our "civilized world." Both mental and physical overexertion often lead first to kidney *qi* vacuity, then to kidney *yang* vacuity, and with prolonged overexertion and stress, finally to kidney *yin* vacuity. Too much work under time pressure, a hasty, unbalanced and insufficient diet, and not enough time for rest and relaxation can weaken kidney energy within weeks or months. If such constant exhaustion is not balanced or taken care of, serious disorders can develop in the course of a few years.

Other negative factors are excessive sexual activity and emotional factors such as fear or a sudden mental shock. All of these can undermine kidney energy. Chronic illness, independent of the organ network involved, always weakens kidney energy eventually, since the kidney is the root of all *yin* and *yang* in the body. Kidney energy decreases physiologically with age. This aging process accelerates when kidney energy is carelessly wasted.

TCM believes that the quality of kidney energy for a new life is determined by the health of the parents at the time of conception. If the parents have weak kidney energy when they conceive, their baby will inherit a constitutional weakness.

Foods that strengthen the kidney network

Fish	Smoked fish, oysters, lobster, salmon, shrimp, tuna
Meat	Game: venison, doves, wild pig
Vegetables	Lentils
Grains	Oats, millet, wheat, black soy beans
Nuts and seeds	Walnuts, black sesame

Kidney *Qi* Vacuity (*Shen Qi Xu*)

This condition is a mild precursor of kidney *yang* vacuity.

Symptoms

Fatigue, easily tired, lethargy, depression, gloomy mood, fears, feeling of weakness with pain in the lumbar region, incontinence, enuresis (bedwetting), reduced libido, frigidity, premature ejaculation.

Therapy

Supplement kidney *qi*

激 • KI-7 • KI-3 • GV-4 • CV-4 + Moxa

Preserve *jing*

Kidney *qi* can be replenished using the same foods as for kidney *yang* vacuity.

Kidney *Yang* Vacuity (*Shen Yang Xu*)

Kidney *yang* vacuity develops from kidney *qi* vacuity.

Kidney *yang* vacuity usually presents with cold symptoms. Since kidney *yang* is the root of all *yang* energies in our body, kidney *yang* vacuity causes extensive cold symptoms in the bowels and viscera (*zang fu* organs), lethargy, and weakness. Digestive disorders of stomach and spleen can result from insufficient warming (symptoms: lack of appetite, sloppy stools). Weak kidney *yang* prevents sufficient warming of *jing*, which weakens energy.

Western diagnosis:
Urological disorders such as chronic cystitis (urinary tract infection), nephritis, prostatitis, urethritis, sexual problems such as frigidity, impotence, and premature ejaculation; depression, anxiety, recurrent lumbago, sciatica, degenerative arthropathy, rheumatoid arthritis, impaired hearing, tinnitus.

Symptoms

General sensitivity to cold, weakness, lethargy, very susceptible to illnesses; sensation of cold and weakness in lower back as well as in knees, coupled with lower back and knee pain. Gloomy mood, depression, withdrawal, fearfulness, frequent urination with clear urine, nycturia (excessive urination at night), incontinence, loss of libido, impotence, frigidity, amenorrhea (lack of menstruation), fertility disorders, hearing loss, dizziness, tinnitus, morning diarrhea, lack of appetite, soft stools.

Therapy

Strengthen kidneys

激 • KI-7 • GV-4 • CV-4 • CV-6 • BL-23 + Moxa

Strengthen *ming men* (life gate)

激 • GV-4 + Moxa

The same dietary recommendations apply to kidney *qi* vacuity and kidney *yang* vacuity.

Avoid

All thermally cool or cold foods, frozen foods, raw foods, thermally cold fruit (e.g., citrus and tropical fruit), salads, sour milk products, excessive consumption of liquids (e.g., mineral water high in sodium) and thermally cold beverages (e.g., orange juice).

The following foods have a strong kidney-energy-weakening effect: Refined sugar and alcoholic beverages, especially high-proof alcohol.

Recommended:

Thermal nature	Moderately hot, warm, neutral foods
Cooking method	Warming
Flavor	Hot–salty, warm–salty, neutral–salty
Fish	Oysters; all smoked fish, especially salmon; mussels, shrimp, tuna
Meat	Especially venison, lamb, wild pig, dove, duck, pork
Vegetables	Fennel, cabbage prepared with warming spices, leeks, radish, root vegetables, onions
Fruit	Cherries, grapes
Beverages	Grain coffee, spiced tea, yogi tea
Grains	Buckwheat, oats, millet, rice (roasted before cooking)
Spices	Ginger, garlic, black pepper, cinnamon
Legumes	Adzuki beans, lentils, black soy beans
Nuts and seeds	Chestnuts, lotus seeds, especially roasted black sesame, sunflower seeds, roasted walnuts

Master Soup with warming types of meat, vegetables, and seasonings.

Thermally hot foods, especially hot seasoning, should not be used excessively, since they can dry out fluids and weaken *yin*. Eating two to three warm meals daily and strengthening the body with kidney-warming foods is advisable, especially for kidney *yang* vacuity. Combining nutritional therapy with foods that strengthen the center burner is recommended.

Comment/Prognosis

TCM considers deficiency or vacuity conditions in the kidney network serious disorders requiring careful treatment. This includes addressing the damaging lifestyle that led to the disorders. Following thorough diagnosis, treatment should include acupuncture and moxibustion, nutritional therapy, Chinese herbs, and movement therapy (*qi gong, tai chi*). Acupuncture treatments should be appropriately supplemented with nutritional therapy. Strengthening and warming foods for the kidneys, prepared using appropriate cooking methods, accelerate treatment success. In conjunction with supplementing kidney energy, nutritional therapy needs to also supplement and sustain the stomach and spleen. Serious disorders such as kidney *yang* vacuity or kidney *yin* vacuity might require Chinese herbal remedies. Depending on the seriousness of the condition, treatment may require weeks to months of consistent therapy. Profound disorders of the kidney network may even require treatment for a number of years. With correct diagnosis and therapy, good to very good results can be achieved. The prognosis is not so good for constitutional kidney *qi* vacuity, essence vacuity, or *jing* vacuity, perhaps caused by massive external damage such as shock or drugs. These are difficult to treat and improvements or modest success often take years to accomplish. Nutritional therapy as well as medicinal herb therapy can significantly strengthen kidney energy, as can a change of circumstances and lifestyle. Kidney *yin* vacuity, or general *yin* vacuity, however, do not respond well, if at all, to acupuncture. These conditions require nutritional and medicinal herb therapy.

Kidney *Yin* Vacuity (*Shen Yin Xu*)

Kidney *yin* vacuity, as a deep disturbance of the kidney network, is associated with essence vacuity (*jing* vacuity), since essence is part of the kidney *yin*.

Kidney *yin* vacuity causes fluid deficiency. Effulgent *yin* vacuity fire (*yin xu huo wang*, or internally developed heat) can form in the body, which further depletes *yin* fluids (symptoms include agitation, redness of the cheeks, dry mouth, and sore throat). One important symptom of *yin* vacuity with vacuity heat is night sweating, also known in TCM as "thief sweating (*yin xu dao han*)," which causes loss of *yin*-nourishing essence. TCM believes that all body fluids, for example blood or sweat, are valuable nourishing substances that need to be preserved. Kidney *yin* vacuity can cause depression, lethargy, mental sluggishness, forgetfulness, and premature aging.

Western diagnosis:
Severe exhaustion, burnout syndrome, chronic consumptive disorders, spermatorrhea (frequent involuntary emission of semen), constitutional weakness, and chronic lumbar spine problems.

Pathogenesis

All factors that cause kidney *qi* or kidney *yang* vacuity and persist over time eventually result in kidney *yin* vacuity. Disease progression is exacerbated by chronic consumptive disorders, protracted fevers, excessive use of drugs and alcohol, heavy blood loss, extreme stress, and chronic sleep deprivation. "Graveyard" shifts, night work

Symptoms

A typical symptom of *yin* vacuity, especially kidney *yin* vacuity, is the above-mentioned night sweat, often accompanied by the five hearts (*wu yi*), or hot areas: hot soles of the feet, hot palms of the hands, heat and burning behind the sternum. Additional symptoms are dry mouth, dry throat, thirst, back and bone pain, tinnitus, hearing loss, dizziness, forgetfulness, impotence, infertility, premature ejaculation, deep and dark rims around the eyes.

Tongue: Red, chapped, no tongue fur
Pulse: Vacuous, rapid, stringlike

Therapy

Enrich kidney *yin*
激 • KI-3 • BL-23 • KI-6 • KI-7 • KI-10

Preserve and support *yin*
激 • CV-4 • SP-6

Avoid:

Warming foods:	
Cooking method	Warming
Flavor	Bitter–hot, bitter–warm, acrid–warm, acrid–hot
Beverages	Coffee, red wine, too much black tea and green tea
Spices	Acrid spices, salt

Also avoid strong mental and physical overexertion, lack of sleep, stress, and excessive sexual activity.

Recommended:

Thermal nature	Neutral, cooling foods that moisten and produce fluids
Cooking method	Cooling
Flavor	Salty–neutral, salty–cool, sweet–neutral, sweet–cool
Meat	Pork, duck, dove
Fish	Oysters, octopus, perch, carp
Fruit	Pears, refreshing fruit, grapes
Vegetables	Refreshing vegetables, cabbage, asparagus, carrots
Grains	Barley, rice, wheat
Nuts and seeds	Black sesame, walnuts
Other	Butter, cream, sheep's and goat's milk

Comment/Prognosis

With kidney *yin* vacuity, all heat factors that can cause *yang* exuberance and prevent regeneration of kidney *yin* need to be strictly avoided. This includes heat from diet, stress, and chronic overexertion. Cooling and moistening foods that build up kidney *yin* and nourish the body are important for treatment. Therapy should encompass acupuncture, as well as nutrition and Chinese herbs. Kidney *yin* vacuity is a profound imbalance that requires several months of therapy to achieve improvements. Nutritional therapy with kidney essence vacuity (*jing* vacuity) can be supportive for kidney essence vacuity (*jing* vacuity) for months or even years. The prognosis for treating *jing* vacuity, however, is unfavorable.

The damaging effect of the bitter–warm drug coffee is often underestimated. Large amounts of coffee (six to eight cups daily) dry up fluids and damage kidney *yin* over time.

Strengthening and enriching kidney *yin* and warming kidney *yang* with appropriate foods supplements the entire *yin* and *yang* of the body. Since all chronic illnesses eventually weaken kidney energy, it is often advisable to address kidney energy in the treatment of a wide variety of disorders.

Kidney *Yin* Vacuity (*Shen Yin Xu*), Heart *Yin* Vacuity (*Xin Yin Xu*), Noninteraction of the Heart and Kidney (*Xin Shen Bu Jiao*)

This syndrome involves a weakening of two important organ networks: kidney *yin* and heart *yin*. The condition, which should be taken very seriously, often appears in times of intense physical and emotional strain and leads patients to see a practitioner with a variety of different symptoms.
When the *yin* of an organ is reduced, especially kidney *yin* as the root of all *yin*, *yang* can no longer be sufficiently contained. Exuberant *yang* produces heat, which further depletes the already weakened *yin*. *Yin* vacuity produces *yang* hyperactivity (*yin xu yang kang*). If heart and kidney *yin* are both weakened, *yang* fire can display distinct symptoms in the area of the spirit (*shen*). Examples are sleep disturbances, heart palpitations, and mental restlessness. This reflects insufficient kidney *yin* for cooling the heart fire. The association between kidney *yin* vacuity and heart *yin* vacuity results from the deep and sensitive *jue yin* (reverting *yin*) axis. TCM believes that when this axis between heart and kidneys is completely severed, the process of dying begins. The negative effects of our modern civilization, such as intense physical strain with inadequate rest, mental stress, financial worries, relationship issues, existential fears, and an unbalanced diet, make this an increasingly common condition.

Western diagnosis:
Deeply exhausted patients, burnout syndrome, chronic consumptive disorders, spermatorrhea (frequent involuntary emission of semen), sexual hyperactivity, irritability, sleep disorders.

Pathogenesis

This symptom complex is rooted in kidney *yin* vacuity and is intensified by extreme emotional strain, such as fear, grief, and depression. Serious emotional impacts, such as the sudden ending of a relationship, can weaken heart *yin* and, when combined with fear, can sever the important deep *jue yin* axis between heart and kidney.

Symptoms

Impotence, fertility disorders, amenorrhea (lack of menstruation), severe exhaustion, dizziness, forgetfulness, sleep disorders, mental restlessness, heart palpitations, lower back pain, nocturnal emissions, erotic dreams, strong sexual desire, back pain, irritability.

Therapy

Enrich kidney *yin* and heart *yin*

• KI-3 • CV-4 • SP-6 • HT-5

Calm *shen*

• HT-7 • GV-20

Clear heart vacuity fire

• HT-6 • PC-8 • PC-7

Avoid:
Thermally hot and warm foods, cooking methods that increase *yang* in foods; high-proof alcoholic beverages, sweets, extreme lifestyles, mental overexertion, sexual excess; stimulating drugs such as amphetamines and ecstasy.

Recommended:

Thermal nature	Neutral, cool and refreshing foods
Cooking method	Cooling
Flavor	Bitter–neutral, bitter–cool, salty–neutral, salty–cool
Meat	Pork, beef, poultry
Fruit	Apples, bananas, refreshing types of fruit
Vegetables	Refreshing types of vegetables, mushrooms, asparagus, spinach, tomatoes
Grains	Barley, wheat germ, rice, corn
Beverages	Lemon balm tea, peppermint tea, wheat beer

Comment/Prognosis

This very serious syndrome requires an immediate change of circumstances, sometimes including psychotherapy. Dietary measures can only play a supplementary role in treating this syndrome, with some relief provided mainly by avoiding warming foods. Quieting *yang* hyperactivity with a combination of acupuncture and Chinese herbs is mandatory. At the same time, the entire body has to be balanced using dietary measures.

Organ Network:
• Liver–Gallbladder
• Wood Phase

Bowel (*Zang* Organ): Liver (*Gan*), LR

Character

"In charge of the Interior"

Loves the unobstructed, harmonious flow of *qi* and thus assures all bodily functions work well. Distinguishes itself by strategic planning.

Role in TCM:

- Governs free coursing of *qi*
- Stores blood (*xue*)
- Stores the ethereal soul (*hun*)
- Governs muscles and sinews
- Governs the making of strategy
- Opens at the eyes and blooms in the nails

Association with the five phases:

- *Emotion*: Rage, anger
- Climate factor: Wind
- *Season*: Spring
- Direction: East
- *Color*: Green
- Time of day: 1–3 a.m.

Viscera (*Fu* Organ): Gallbladder (*Dan*), GB

Character

"The Official who Makes Decisions"

Function

- Supports digestion
- Looks after the "inner plan for life"
- Gives courage and initiative
- Time of day: 11 p.m.–1 a.m.

Organ Network Liver–Gallbladder

• Governs free coursing of *qi*

The most important function of the liver is to ensure unobstructed and uninterrupted *qi* flow in the body by coordinating and controlling the amount and speed of coursing *qi* and substances. This requires equilibrium and harmony. Emotional impacts such as anger and rage immediately block *qi* flow (liver *qi* stagnation).

Symptoms

Muscle tension, feeling of oppression, chest tightness, premenstrual syndrome, and abdominal distension.

• Stores blood (*xue*)

Another function of the liver is the storage of blood (*xue*). During periods of rest, when lying down or sleeping, blood flows to the liver, is retained there and then regenerated. The spleen network is responsible for the production of blood, while the heart network keeps the blood flowing.

Emotions such as anger or rage seriously impact the flow of *qi* and can easily block or obstruct *qi* flow. Protracted unresolved obstructions lead to development of internal heat from such "heated emotions," causing symptoms such as ascendant liver *yang* (*gan yang shang kang*), liver fire (*gan huo shang yan*), depletion of liver *yin*, and liver wind (*gan feng*).

Nutrition and Organ Network

The sour flavor associated with the liver is astringent and contracting, which gathers body fluids and protects blood. Unhealthy eating habits, strong emotions such as aggression, anger, and rage, and a hectic and stressful lifestyle produce liver heat and impair liver function.

- Diet, especially spices and alcohol, can help disperse *qi* obstruction to some extent, but its impact is limited. Acupuncture, Chinese herbs, and movement therapy are more appropriate treatments.
- With liver heat, it is absolutely necessary to reduce energetically hot foods and emphasize cooling foods.
- With blood and liver *yin* vacuity, strengthen blood and *yin* via the liver network.
- Anger, rage, and heated emotions can be "calmed" or drained by cooling foods.

Liver Syndromes and Chinese Nutrition

Binding depression of liver *qi* (stagnation) (*gan qi yu jie*)
Ascendant liver *yang* (*gan yang shang kang*)
Liver fire flaming upward (*gan huo shang yan*)
Liver *yin* vacuity (*gan yin xu*)
Liver blood vacuity (*gan xue xu*)

Imbalances of the liver network are very common. The primary purpose of this network is to smooth and regulate the coursing of *qi*. The liver is the most important organ for the preservation of blood. Large amounts of blood return to the liver at night and are regenerated there. The liver opens at the eyes, which can show signs of possible imbalances.

Western diagnosis:
Temporal headache, hypertension, sleep disorders, gynecological problems such as dysmenorrhea (painful menstrual cramps) and premenstrual syndrome (PMS). Emotional imbalance with irritability and aggression.

Causes

Diet: Warming foods and cooking methods, especially acrid spices, high-proof alcohol, and very fatty or oily foods, can damage the liver. They have a heating effect and thus "ignite" liver *yang*, which in turn damages liver *yin*. This often results in ascending liver *yang*, or, in its more extreme form, liver fire flaming upward (*gan huo shang yan*), which is often accompanied by liver *yin* vacuity. In women, liver *yin* vacuity frequently presents as blood vacuity.

General: The liver is sensitive to external pathogenic factors such as wind and dampness and especially sensitive to emotional upsets. Chinese medicine views the liver as a filter for all emotional impact. The liver distributes the impact in the body. Anger, rage, and resentment cause the liver to "cramp up" and inhibit the smooth coursing of *qi*. One of the most common syndromes in clinical practice is binding depression of liver *qi* (*gan qi yu jie*), which is mainly attributable to emotional imbalance. Even small emotional impacts such as arguments, frustrations, etc. can block liver *qi*. Over a period of time (months to years) these problems accumulate and root deeply inside the body. In addition to "undigested" emotions, a hectic and stressful lifestyle can also overheat the liver.

! Restoring balance to the liver network requires not only dietary changes, but also changes in lifestyle, such as stress reduction, regular relaxation exercises, rest and meditation periods, as well as appropriate expression of one's emotions.

Binding Depression of Liver *Qi* (*Gan Qi Yu Jie*)

Western diagnosis:
Menstrual disorders, gynecological problems such as dysmenorrhea (painful menstrual cramps), disorders of the vegetative (autonomous) nervous system, premenstrual syndrome, depression.

Symptoms

Feeling of congestion and swelling in chest, bloating in epigastric region, gas, irritability, depression, frustrations, mood swings with sudden outbursts of feeling, impaired appetite, premenstrual syndrome (PMS), nausea, retching, stomach aches, diarrhea (restraining cycle, or *xiang ke*—liver excess attacks the stomach).

Tongue: Vividly colored, curled at the edges

Pulse: Tight

Therapy

Clear binding depression of liver *qi*
激 • LR-3 • LR-14 • GB-34 • LR-13

Avoid:
Foods that burden the liver.

Beverages	Alcohol, coffee
Other	Drugs, food coloring, preservatives, heavily spiced foods, sugar

Recommended:
Only a few foods have a calming effect on the liver.

Fruit	Plums
Vegetables	Radish, Chinese leek (garlic chives), celery, brown seaweed
Nuts and seeds	Black sesame
Other	Crayfish, prawns (shrimp), vinegar

To stimulate *qi* flow

Flavor	Mild–acrid
Spices	Ginger, garlic, pepper (these spices should be used only in small amounts, otherwise they can damage the liver), marjoram
Vegetables	Kohlrabi, leeks, radish
Other	Alcohol, coriander, chili (careful, hot!)

Binding depression of liver *qi is* commonly found in practice with different levels of intensity. It is very well suited for acupuncture treatment, but is also suitable for treatment with Chinese phytotherapy. Acupuncture treatments such as the combination LI-4 Union Valley (*he gu*) and LR-3 Supreme Surge (*tai chong*) are very useful in dissolving binding depression of liver *qi*.

■ Ascendant Liver *Yang* (*Gan Yang Shang Kang*)

Western diagnosis:
Cephalgia (headaches), hypertension (high blood pressure), migraine, vertigo, conjunctivitis, glaucoma, Ménière disease (auditory vertigo), tinnitus.

Symptoms
Irritability, loss of temper, temporal headaches, feelings of pressure behind the eyes, vertigo (dizziness), tinnitus, hearing loss, sleep disorders, dry mouth.

Tongue: Red, especially at the edges

Pulse: Stringlike, tight

Causes

Diet: Highly warming foods such as alcohol and acrid spices, as well as cooking methods that increase *yang* produce heat and cause *yang* to ascend. This also weakens liver *yin*. An excess of fatty foods and oils obstructs the coursing of *qi* and this stagnation can cause heat.

General: Emotional impact such as suppressed anger, rage, resentment, or frustrations are the most common causes for ascending liver *yang*. Liver *yin* vacuity or kidney *yin* vacuity can also cause ascending liver *yang*. Excessive lifestyles, emotional imbalance, frustration, living with constant time pressure, and unhealthy eating habits are witnessed more and more often in practice. These can cause a multitude of ailments such as upper burner disorders, tinnitus, headaches, dizziness, and sleep disorders.

Therapy

Strengthen liver *yang*
激 • LR-8 • SP-6 • KI-3

Clear heat
激 • LR-2 • LR-3

Drain *yang*
激 • LR-3 • GB-20 • GB-34 • GV-20

Avoid

Thermal nature	Warm and hot foods
Cooking method	Warming
Flavor	Bitter–hot, bitter–warm, acrid–warm, acrid–hot, sweet–hot, salty–hot, and sour–hot
Spices	Acrid spices, ginger, garlic, pepper, chili
Beverages	High-proof alcohol, coffee
Other	Food coloring, preservatives, salt, very oily and fatty foods, sugar

Tip: No meat for six weeks!

Recommended:

All foods that have downbearing movement and enrich *yin*.

Thermal nature	Neutral–cool, cold foods
Cooking method	Cooling, raw foods
Flavor	Sour–cool, sour–cold, bitter–cool, bitter–cold
Fruit	Rhubarb, lemons, apples, mangos, mulberry fruit
Vegetables	Spinach, sprouts, tomatoes, raw vegetables, dandelion, gentian, Belgian endive hearts, celery
Beverages	Green tea, peppermint tea, wheat beer, bread drink (a lacto-fermented beverage made from grain), apple juice
Grains	Spelt, wheat, wheat germ, mung beans, mung bean sprouts
Dairy products	Sour milk products, yogurt
Legumes	Mung beans, mung bean sprouts
Other	Salt

Despite its alcohol content, wheat beer is very cooling for the liver and enriches *yin*.

Comment/Prognosis

With ascendant liver *yang*, all heat-generating foods should be avoided. Treatment should begin with a cooling and *yin* enriching diet (four to six weeks of only vegetarian foods). In addition to acupuncture treatment, supplemented with Chinese herbs, it is important to convey to the patient that long-term stabilization requires a change in lifestyle (no stress, no anger!). With TCM as adjunct therapy, good to very good results can be obtained, depending on the changes made. Physical exercise outdoors is important!

Liver Fire Flaming Upward (*Gan Huo Shang Yan*)

Western diagnosis:
Cephalgia (headaches), migraine, hypertension (high blood pressure), Ménière disease (auditory vertigo), tinnitus, chronic conjunctivitis.

Symptoms

Restlessness, insomnia, irritability, sudden loss of temper, vertigo (dizziness), severe headaches, red eyes, intraocular pressure, dry mouth, bitter taste in mouth, nose bleeds, tinnitus.

Tongue: Dry, red, red edges, yellow fur
Pulse: Tight, rapid

Causes

Diet: Excess alcohol, overly spicy and overly fatty foods. Overuse of warming cooking methods such as grilling, barbecuing, searing, frying, etc.

General: Common cause is liver *qi* stagnation resulting from prolonged emotional disharmony, such as anger, frustration, and rage.

Therapy

Cool liver fire
激 • LR-2 • LR-3 • GB-20
• GB-34 • LR-8 • GB-13

Avoid:

Thermal nature	Hot and warm foods
Cooking method	Warming
Flavor	Acrid–hot, acrid–warm, salty–hot, sweet–hot, bitter–hot, sour–hot
Foods	High-proof alcohol, strongly seasoned foods, very fatty and very oily foods

Recommended:

Thermal nature	Cool and cold foods
Cooking method	Cooling, raw foods
Flavor	Sour–cool, sour–cold, bitter–cool, bitter–cold
Foods	Reduce salt and meat, vegetarian diet for several days or weeks, no alcohol, no sugar, no coffee; see also dietary recommendations for ascending liver yang, page 93.

With liver fire flaming upward, choose foods with a downbearing and strongly cooling effect.

Fruit	Bananas, rhubarb, watermelons, lemons, tropical fruits
Vegetables	Cucumbers, water chestnuts, spinach, tomatoes, celery
Beverages	Yerba mate tea, wheat beer, vermouth
Dairy products	Yogurt
Other	Salt, dandelion, gentian

Comment/Prognosis

With this syndrome, all heating foods need to be strictly avoided. Symptoms often appear suddenly, and immediate acupuncture can help manage them. Combined with Chinese herbal remedies, long-term treatment can achieve good results.

Liver *Yin* Vacuity (*Gan Yin Xu*)

Liver *yin* vacuity rarely occurs as a single syndrome. It is often combined with the following syndromes: ascending liver *yang*, liver fire flaming upward, and blood or liver blood vacuity.

Western diagnosis:
Hypertension (high blood pressure), chronic conjunctivitis, cephalgia (headaches), and chronic migraine

Symptoms

Nervousness, internal restlessness, dry eyes, vertigo (dizziness), headaches, red face, red cheeks, hot palms and soles of feet (typical sign of *yin* vacuity), impaired vision, depression.

Tongue: Reddish, dry
Pulse: Thin, rapid, stringlike

Causes

Diet: Overly acrid foods, overuse of cooking methods that increase *yang*, too many fatty, oily foods.

General: Extreme physical and emotional strain can weaken liver *yin*. Excessive night work weakens liver *yin* and also blood since, according to TCM, blood is stored and regenerated in the liver at night. This syndrome is becoming more and more common, since long hours in front of the computer weaken liver *yin*.

Excess *yang* energy, for example due to heated emotional strain or hot foods, provokes syndromes such as ascending liver *yang* or liver fire.

Therapy

Nourish liver *yin*
激 • LR-8 • SP-6 • KI-3 • BL-18

Avoid:

Thermal nature	Hot and warm foods
Flavor	Bitter–hot, acrid–hot, sour–hot
Cooking method	Warming
Foods	All foods that further weaken yin, especially acrid spices, coffee, high-proof alcohol, red wine, smoking

Recommended:

Thermal nature	Cool, cold, and neutral foods
Cooking method	Cooling
Flavor	Sour–refreshing, sour–cool, sour–neutral, sweet–cool, sweet–cold
Vegetables	Cucumbers, sauerkraut, celeriac (celery root), spinach, tomatoes
Beverages	Bread drink (a lacto-fermented beverage made from grain)
Grains	Spelt, barley, wheat
Dairy products	Sour milk products
Soy products	Tofu

Comment/Prognosis

A balanced diet with neutral and slightly cooling foods, as well as avoiding excess of warming foods, along with other lifestyle changes can improve symptoms.

■ Liver Blood Vacuity (*Gan Xue Xu*)

This symptom usually appears in combination with liver *yin* vacuity.

Western diagnosis:
Anemia, neuroses, menstrual disorders such as dysmenorrhea, amenorrhea.

Symptoms

Vertigo (dizziness), blurred vision, dry eyes, dull complexion, pronounced paleness, night blindness, general weakness, numbness of extremities, tremors, cramps, menstrual disorders such as amenorrhea, insomnia.

Causes

Diet: An excess of overly spicy and warming foods weaken body *yin*. Foods that are too cold reduce spleen *qi* and inhibit the formation of blood.

General: Blood loss, for example during surgery or childbirth. Exaggerated activity at night, when the liver stores and regenerates blood. Blood is an important *yin* substance that is built up primarily by good spleen function, but also by good kidney function. Prolonged negative impacts on the three organs spleen, kidney, and liver result in blood vacuity. Since blood is the mode of transportation for *qi*, blood vacuity weakens the entire body. Sinew, muscle, and nail problems result from malnutrition caused by blood vacuity. Blood is the "bed of rest" for the spirit (*shen*), which cannot be firmly anchored with liver blood vacuity. Symptoms include insomnia, sleepwalking, and mental instability.

Therapy

Generate liver blood

激 • SP-10 • SP-6 • BL-17 • BL-18 • LR-8

Enrich kidney *yin*

激 • KI-3 • KI-6 • SP-6

Supplement spleen *qi*

激 • SP-3 • BL-20 • BL-21

Avoid:

Warming cooking methods, thermally hot foods. All bitter foods, especially the flavors bitter–hot and bitter–warm. Acrid–hot and acrid–warm flavors, since these dry out blood. Black tea, cocoa, acrid spices, such as garlic, ginger, pepper, curry, cinnamon, etc. Energetically hot beverages such as **coffee**, high-proof alcohol, yogi tea.

Recommended:

Cooking method	Cooling
Flavors	Sweet–neutral, sweet–warm, sour–neutral, sour–cool
Grains	Amaranth, short-grain (glutinous) rice, rice
Vegetables	All thermally neutral and refreshing vegetables, especially those of a red color such as beets, red cabbage, carrots, as well as spinach, fennel
Meat	Poultry, poultry liver, beef, beef stock, beef liver, veal liver, lamb liver (liver preferably from organically raised animals)
Fish	Oysters, mussels, octopus, perch, eel
Fruit	Red types of fruit such as grapes, sweet cherries, longans (a type of lychee), plums
Nuts and seeds	Sesame, sunflower seeds
Beverages	Red beet juice, sweet cherry juice, plum juice, red tea (rosehip tea, hibiscus), red grape juice, red wine in moderation

Recommended for liver blood vacuity:

Meat	Poultry, duck, rabbit liver, hare liver, pork liver (liver preferably from organically raised animals)
Fish	Oysters, crab, white fish, perch
Fruit	Apples, lychees, plums, grapes, longans (a type of lychee)
Vegetables	Thermally neutral and cooling vegetables from the wood phase that are green in color, such as beans, broccoli, lamb's lettuce, lotus root, mangold chard, spinach, sprouts, tomatoes
Beverages	Carrot juice, tomato juice
Grains	Wheat, short-grain (glutinous) rice
Spices	Watercress, marjoram, parsley root
Nuts and seeds	Sesame, sunflower seeds
Other	Egg yolk

Organ Network:
• Heart–Small Intestine
• Fire Phase

Bowel (*Zang* Organ): Heart (*Xin*), HT

Character

"Ruler and Godlike Emperor"

The heart represents all the emotional, mental, and spiritual abilities and activities that make up the unique personality of a person. It is the seat of consciousness and mental vitality.

Role in TCM:

- Governs blood (*xue*) and blood vessels
- Governs circulation of blood
- Houses spirit (*shen*)
- Opens at the tongue and governs speech, sense of taste

Association with the five phases:

- Emotion: Joy
- Climate factor: Heat
- *Season:* Summer
- Direction: South
- Color: Red
- Flavor: Bitter
- *Time of day:* 11 a.m.–1 p.m.

Viscera (*Fu* Organ): Small Intestine (*Xiao Chang*)

Character

"Holds the Office of Reception"

Function

- Receives "water and grain" (food) that has been decomposed in the stomach and transforms it further.
- Separates the turbid from the clear liquids and extracts nutrients from food.
- On a mental level: Facilitates powers of judgment and distinction between important and unimportant
- Time of day: 1–3 p.m.

Organ Network Heart–Small Intestine

- **Houses spirit (*shen*)**

Shen comprises spirit or "consciousness" in its broadest sense: The mental, intellectual, emotional and spiritual abilities of a person. TCM believes that these are closely connected to heart, blood, and *yin*. Blood is a material anchor for *shen*. Disturbances of the spirit (insomnia or confusion; *shen pi*, or lassitude of spirit and lack of strength) can be associated with material aspects such as heart blood vacuity. The spirit can be calmed by avoiding energetically very hot foods (garlic, ginger, alcohol). Often these dietary measures are in keeping with religious or spiritual dietary recommendations intended to calm the mind. Strengthening blood can cure certain types of insomnia.

- **Governs blood**

The heart is responsible for anchoring *qi* extracted from food (*gu qi*) in the blood and for circulation of blood in the body.

Nutrition and Organ Network

- An excess of hot foods should be avoided to keep the spirit and heart calm.
- Avoid further stimulating external heat (climate factor) or "inner" heat resulting from stress and frenzy or from drinking coffee or eating acrid spices.
- An excess of bitter flavors can dry out blood and body fluids.
- Building up heart *yin* through dietary measures can support blood.
- Blood stagnation, similar to *qi* stagnation, can only be partially resolved through dietary measures, and is more successfully treated with acupuncture and Chinese herbs.

Heart Syndromes and Chinese Nutrition

Heart *qi* vacuity (*xin qi xu*)
Heart *yang* vacuity (*xin yan xu*)
Heart blood vacuity (*xin xue xu*)
Heart *yin* vacuity (*xin jin xu*)
Heart fire flaming upward (*xin huo shang yan*)

TCM believes the heart to be the emperor of the body. Its most important function is to house the spirit (*shen*). The spirit resides in blood and *yin*, creating a natural connection between heart and blood. Besides the mental and spiritual connection, the heart (fire phase) warms the body and provides it with liveliness. Joy is associated with the heart. Other important functions of the heart network are to govern blood (*xue*) and blood vessels and to govern sweat. Disharmonies in the heart network are caused by emotions such as extreme joy, but also by sadness and anger. Other triggering factors for heart problems can be a heavy workload under intense time pressure; external pathogenic factors, especially heat; and lack of joy or love.

Western diagnosis:
Insomnia, restlessness, heart palpitations, paroxysmal tachycardia, tachyarrhythmia, vertigo (dizziness), night sweats, nightmares, cardiovascular disorders.

Therapy

General: Dietary treatments for disharmonies in the heart network are limited. As with all repletion (excess) syndromes that display heat symptoms, avoiding *yang* foods and cooking methods and giving preference to soothing *yin* products and cooling cooking methods is recommended. Vacuity patterns can be treated with warm and neutral foods. Bitter–warm and bitter–neutral flavors of the fire phase are recommended.

The heart network is especially sensitive to external and internal heat. In treating heart disharmony conditions, overly hot and warm foods such as acrid spices or high-proof alcohol should be used very sparingly. Even small amounts of acrid foods, for example pepper or garlic eaten in the late evening, can cause sleep disturbance, restlessness, etc.

The syndrome "heart fire flaming upward" (*xin huo shang yan*) should be treated by restricting all *yang* foods and cooking methods and by using bitter–cool foods. The syndromes "phlegm–fire harassing the heart" (*tan huo rao xin*) and "phlegm confounding the orifices of the heart" (*tan mi xin qiao*) should be treated by following the dietary recommendations for reducing phlegm and by making use of phlegm-loosening foods. These conditions are more successfully treated with herbal remedies and acupuncture. The same holds true for "heart blood stasis obstruction." Chinese nutrition is effective for treating the following syndromes: heart *yang* vacuity, heart blood vacuity, and heart *yin* vacuity.

■ Heart *Yang* Vacuity (*Xin Yang Xu*)

Heart *qi* vacuity and heart *yang* vacuity are treated with the same nutritional therapy. Heart *yang* vacuity, with its additional cold component, differs in its symptoms from heart *qi* vacuity.

Western diagnosis:
Autonomic heart conditions, convalescence, cardiac arrhythmia, exhaustion.

Symptoms

Listlessness, fatigue, exhaustion, cold extremities, pale glowing face, dyspnea (shortness of breath) on exertion, chest tightness in the area of the heart, sometimes racing heart with sensation of extreme heart beats, shortness of breath, spontaneous sweating.

Tongue: Pale, slightly swollen
Pulse: Weak

Causes

General: Extreme emotional strain, especially sadness, can first cause heart *qi* vacuity and then heart *yang* vacuity. Blood loss first weakens heart *qi* and then heart *yang*. Heart *yang* vacuity can also be partially caused by kidney *yang* vacuity, since the kidneys are the root of *yang* in the body. Symptoms appear in the periphery of the body, the head, and the extremities, since the body no longer has sufficient *yang* energy to adequately supply these areas.

Therapy

Strengthen and supplement heart *yang*
Supplement *yang*

激 • HT-5 • BL-15 • CV-4 • CV-6 • Moxa

Avoid:
All foods that reduce and weaken *yang*.

Thermal nature	All cool and cold foods
Cooking method	Cooling
Flavor	Bitter–cool, bitter–cold
Vegetables	Raw vegetables
Fruit	Citrus fruits
Dairy products	Yogurt
Other	Ice cream, ice-cold drinks; also frozen foods and foods heated in the microwave, since they do not have sufficient qi.

Recommended:

Thermal nature	Warm–neutral; hot in small amounts
Cooking method	Warming
Flavor	Bitter–warm; bitter–hot in moderation, sour–hot/warm, sweet–hot/warm, acrid–hot/warm
Meat	Lamb, beef
Grains	Buckwheat, corn, short-grain (glutinous) rice, oats
Beverages	Yogi tea, warm wheat beer, coffee, cocoa
Other	Aniseed, chili

! Coffee dries up blood and should be consumed only in moderation, despite its bitter–hot effect; if possible, add warming spices such as cardamom or cinnamon to reduce the stagnation-causing effects of coffee.

Comment/Prognosis

Lifestyle changes such as going to sleep before 11 p.m. and sufficient rest and relaxation periods are important. Heart *yang* and heart *qi* can be regenerated within weeks or months with longer periods of rest and by following the appropriate dietary recommendations.

■ Heart Blood Vacuity (*Xin Xue Xu*)

Western Diagnoses:
Anemia, autonomic heart conditions, exhaustion, and convalescence.

Symptoms

Pale face, pale lips, heart palpitations, fatigue, weakness, inner restlessness, forgetfulness, easily startled, frequent blinking, sleep disturbance with many dreams, vertigo (dizziness), trouble falling asleep, nightmares, depression, agitation.

Tongue: Pale, tear in the center, sometimes swelling at the tip

Pulse: Thin

Causes

Diet: Overly acrid foods that damage *yin*. Highly dehydrating foods such as coffee or alcohol. Dietary errors that cause spleen vacuity and prevent sufficient blood formation.

General: Heart blood vacuity generally has the same causes as general blood vacuity or liver blood acuity. Loss of blood, for example during childbirth, too much stress, extreme physical activity (sweating weakens *qi* and *yang* energy), lingering emotional problems, especially sadness and anger, all damage *yin*.

Therapy

Strengthen heart blood
激 • BL-15 • CV-14 • CV-15

Supplement spleen
激 • SP-6 • BL-20 • ST-36 • SP-3

Enrich body *yin*
激 • SP-6 • KI-6 • KI-3 • CV-4

Avoid:

Thermal nature	Foods that are too hot or too warm
Cooking method	Warming
Foods	Highly dehydrating foods such as coffee, red wine, acrid spices

Recommended:

Thermal nature	Neutral–warm, cool
Flavor	Sweet–warm, sweet–neutral, sour–neutral
Meat	Blood sausage, chicken meat, beef, pheasant
Fish	Oysters
Fruit	Cherries, longans (a type of lychee), red grapes
Grains	Short-grain (glutinous) rice, wheat, oats
Beverages	Goat's milk, sheep's milk, cow's milk

Also all foods recommended for general strengthening of blood (see p. 60ff.).

Heart *Yin* Vacuity (*Xin Yin Xu*)

Western diagnosis:
Anemia, chronic exhaustion, hypertension (high blood pressure), menopause, chronic sleep disturbances.

Symptoms

Inner restlessness, anxiety, trouble falling asleep with many dreams, trouble sleeping through the night, thirst, dry mouth, agitation, red cheeks, subfebrile (below normal) body temperature in the evening. Especially important differential symptom: Night sweat, hot flushes, hot feet and soles of feet.

Tongue: Red, no fur, red dots at the tip, tear at the tip

Pulse: Vacuous, floating, rapid

Causes

General: Fever, too much talking, stress, always "being on the run," hectic lifestyle, excessive sexual activity late at night.

Differential Diagnosis

Differentiating heart *yang* vacuity from heart *yin* vacuity: Increased trouble sleeping through the night with heart *yin* vacuity; common in middle-aged and older people.

Therapy

Strengthen heart *yin*
激 • HT-6

Calm spirit (*shen*)
激 • GV-20 • CV-15

Enrich body *yin*
激 • SP-6 • KI-6 • KI-3

Avoid:

Thermal nature	Hot and warm foods
Cooking method	Warming
Flavor	Acrid–hot, acrid–warm, bitter–hot, bitter–warm
Foods	All drying and warming foods

Recommended:

Thermal nature	Neutral, cooling, possibly slightly warming foods
Flavor	Sweet–neutral, sweet–warm, sweet–cool, bitter–neutral, sour–neutral, sour–cool
Meat	Beef, (pork)
Fruit	Red grapes
Grains	Wheat (pasta)
Dairy products	Goat's milk cheese, sheep's milk cheese
Nuts and seeds	Poppy seed, black sesame
Other	Poppy seed pastry

■ Heart Fire Flaming Upward (*Xin Huo Shang Yan*)

Western diagnosis:
High blood pressure, autonomic heart conditions, glossitis (burning tongue).

Symptoms

Intense emotional symptoms such as inner restlessness, anxiety, sleep disorders with nightmares, emotional instability and impulsiveness, red face, erosion and ulceration in the mouth area (canker sores), bitter taste in mouth, dark urine.

Tongue: Red tip, yellow fur, red dots
Pulse: Rapid, strong

Causes

Diet: Too many overly spicy and warming foods.

General: Strong emotional agitation and strain, such as long-suppressed fears and worries can suddenly discharge as heart fire flaming upward.

Heart fire flaming upward is frequently associated with kidney *yin* and heart *yin* vacuity, resulting in loss of governance of heart *yang*.

Therapy

Cool heart fire
激 • HT-7 • HT-8 • PC-5

Calm spirit (*shen*)
激 • GV-20 • HT-9

Avoid:

Thermal nature	Warming foods and cooking methods
Flavor	Bitter–hot, acrid–hot
Foods	High-proof alcohol, acrid spices

Recommended:

Thermal nature	Cool and cold foods
Flavor	Bitter–cool, bitter–cold, sour–cool, sour–cold
Fruit	Rhubarb, watermelons, lemons
Vegetables	Raw vegetable salads, tomatoes, dandelion
Beverages	Bread drink (a lacto-fermented beverage made from grain), black tea
Dairy products	Sour milk products
Other	Gentian, vermouth, green tea

Comment/Prognosis

In its acute stage, this syndrome can be only marginally improved through dietary therapy. It can, however, benefit from nutritional therapy in the long term. Treatment should focus on acupuncture and Chinese herbal remedies.

4 Food Classification

Vegetables

Vegetables represent all flavors and all variations of thermal nature. Chinese dietetics believes vegetables to be the ideal complement to grains. The classic *Su Wen* states: "The five types of grain nourish, the five types of vegetables complete."

- To treat **repletion** (robust person; loud, powerful voice; sensation of heat, hyperactivity, choleric features, extroverted, tongue with thick fur, replete pulse): Celery root (celeriac), lettuce, spinach, eggplant, and tomato.
- To treat **vacuity** (weak person; weak, quiet voice; shivering, frequently tired and exhausted, introverted, swollen tongue, weak pulse): Fennel, sweet potatoes, potatoes, carrots, and cabbage.
- To treat **heat** (red face, thirst for cold drinks, worsening of condition and pain with heat, red tongue, rapid pulse): Tomato, cucumber, sprouts (bamboo, soy bean, mung bean), and dandelion.
- To treat **cold** (shivering, aversion to cold, condition and pain worsens with cold, pale, swollen tongue; weak, slow pulse): Leek, onion, green onion, fennel, and carrots.
- To treat **dampness** (general feeling of heaviness, pathological swelling and edema; chronic phlegm disorders, for example frontal sinusitis, bronchitis, cysts, tumors): Belgian endive hearts.
- To treat **dryness** (dry mouth and lips, chapped skin, dry mucous membranes): Tomato, cucumber.

Bamboo Sprouts

Flavor	Sweet
Organ network	Stomach, lung
Direction	Downbearing
Phase	Earth
Effect	Clear heat, enrich *yin*, calm restlessness, transform phlegm, downbear *qi*, diuretic and laxative
Preparation methods	As salad, cold, boiled, stir-fried, or as decoction
Contains	Plenty of water, protein, fat, calcium, phosphorus, potassium, vitamins B_1, B_2, niacin

Indications

- *Heat in stomach:*
  Heartburn, gastritis, ulceration in stomach and intestinal tract, thirst, dry mouth
- *Heat phlegm disorders of the lung:*
  Bronchitis, sinusitis with viscous, yellow phlegm

Boil fresh bamboo sprouts and eat them cold, mixed with a little ginger, salt, and vinegar.

Cabbage

Thermal nature	Neutral
Flavor	Sweet
Organ network	Large intestine, stomach
Direction	Upbearing
Phase	Earth
Effect	Supplements center burner, alleviates acute pain, promotes digestion
Preparation methods	Raw, as salad, or as a juice (good for intestinal ulcers)
Contains	High in vitamin B_1, B_2, C, and A, beta-carotene, flavonoids, calcium, phosphorus, potassium, iron, zinc

Indications

- *Stomach and spleen disharmony and stagnation:* Cramplike-pain in center abdomen, constipation
- Stomach and duodenal ulcers (Western and Chinese medicine views converge here)

Chinese Cabbage (Napa Cabbage)

Thermal nature	Neutral, tendency towards cold
Flavor	Sweet
Organ network	Stomach, large intestine
Direction	Downbearing
Phase	Earth
Effect	Clears heat, promotes digestion, creates body fluids, diuretic and laxative
Preparation methods	Juiced, boiled, or as decoction
Contains	Rich in vitamin A, B_1, and C, niacin, calcium and iron; beta-carotene, magnesium, phosphorus, essential amino acids, mustard oils

Indications

- *Heat in stomach:*
  Gastritis, gastric ulcers, duodenal ulcers, thirst, dry mouth
- *Heat in lung:*
  Feverish cold, cough

Decoction of Chinese cabbage juice, radish, and honey.

- *Dryness and heat in intestine:*
  Constipation, flatulence

Cucumber

Thermal nature	Cool
Flavor	Sweet
Organ network	Spleen, stomach, large intestine
Direction	Downbearing
Phase	Earth
Effect	Clears heat, drains yang, diuretic, reduces swelling, detoxifies, clears skin
Preparation methods	As salad, raw, boiled, fried, or as decoction
Contains	Water, vitamin B_1, B_2, niacin, beta-carotene, rutin, high in potassium, magnesium, amaroids (bitters)

Indications

- *General heat symptoms:*
  Thirst, anxiety, swelling and pain in throat, hoarseness, reddened and swollen eyes, acne, skin inflammations
- *Summer heat:*
  Good nutritional supplement during hot season, especially for conditions brought on by external heat
- *External use:*
  Red, inflamed, swollen and dry eyes; for regeneration of facial skin (in Arabia, cucumber juice was a common ingredient in facial soaps), for first-degree skin burns (sunburn)
- *Damp–heat in large intestine:*
  Traveler's diarrhea

Contraindications

- *Cold and vacuity symptoms in center burner:*
  Stomach aches and diarrhea; worsens with cold

Eggplant (Aubergine)

Thermal nature	Cool
Flavor	Sweet
Organ network	Stomach and spleen, large intestine
Direction	Downbearing
Phase	Earth
Effect	Clears heat, moves and cools blood, disperses blood stasis, reduces swelling, eases pain; harmonizes liver and uterus, especially with suppressed emotions
Preparation methods	Boiled, stir-fried, baked, as juice, decoction or preserved in wine
Contains	Water, carbohydrates, vitamin C, calcium, niacin, iron, phosphorus, above-average amount of potassium, amaroids (bitters), essential oils

Indications

- *Heat in blood:*
  Skin disorders with itching and red cutaneous efflorescence, skin ulcers and growths, breast inflammation (mastitis), carbuncle (external use), bloody stool, hemorrhoids

Green Onions (Spring Onions)

Thermal nature	Warm
Flavor	Acrid
Organ network	Lung, stomach
Direction	Upbearing
Phase	Metal
Effect	Removes external pathogenic weather factors from body surface, moves yang and dissipates cold, detoxifies
Preparation methods	Decoction, juice, paste, stir-fried, steamed or as a spice; decreasing effect when cooked too long.
Contains	Rich in essential oils, predominantly allicin; rich in vitamin C and A, calcium; also vitamin B_1 and B_2; potassium, phosphorus, iron, iodine, and selenium

Indications

- *Colds due to external wind and cold influences:* Shivering, dislike of cold, fever without sweating, headaches, stuffy nose
- *Cold symptoms in center burner:* Abdominal pain and diarrhea

Decoction of green onions and ginger.

- Abdominal pain due to parasite infestation

About 30 g (one tablespoon) each of green onion juice and sesame oil daily.

- Acute ulceration or lesions in the initial stage

Two to three tablespoons of green onion juice with a little brown sugar to taste and hot water; take once daily.

Contraindications

- General lack of strength and tendency to spontaneous sweating

Leek

Thermal nature	Warm
Flavor	Acrid
Organ network	Lung, liver, stomach, kidney
Direction	Upbearing and downbearing
Phase	Wood, metal
Effect	Regulates and moves *qi*, dissolves blood stasis, supplements, supports kidney yang, warms center burner, dissipates cold, disperses wind–cold influences, detoxifies
Contains	Vitamin B_1, rich in vitamin C, iron, magnesium, calcium, phosphorus, amaroids (bitters)

Indications

- *Cold symptoms in center burner:* Dysphagia (difficulty or pain when swallowing), abdominal pain, reduced appetite, diarrhea
- *Kidney yang vacuity:* Loss of libido, impotence, premature ejaculation, back (lumbar) pain, urorrhea (passage of urine per rectum), weakness in back and legs
- *Blood stasis:* Abdominal swelling and pain
- *External wind–cold influences:* First signs of a beginning cold, influenza with chills, aversion to cold

Contraindications

- *Heat symptoms*
- *General yin vacuity*

Lettuce

Thermal nature	Cool
Flavor	Sweet, bitter
Organ network	Large intestine, stomach
Direction	Downbearing
Phase	Fire, earth
Effect	Clears heat, diuretic, stimulates milk flow
Preparation methods	Raw, boiled, or as decoction
Contains	Calcium, vitamin A and C, chlorophyll (stored primarily in outer leaves)

Indications

- *General heat symptoms and heat in bladder:* Restlessness, thirst, nervousness, micturition (urination) problems, burning sensation when urinating; sparse, dark urine
- Disturbance of milk flow after birth

Lotus Root

Thermal nature	Raw: cool Cooked: warming
Flavor	Sweet
Organ network	Stomach, spleen, heart
Direction	Downbearing
Phase	Earth
Effect	When eaten raw, clears heat, produces fluids, cools blood, disperses stagnation; when cooked, supports the center burner, supplements blood, relieves diarrhea.

Indications

- *Heat symptoms:* Fever, thirst, restlessness

Raw lotus root

- *Blood heat symptoms*: Nosebleeds, bloody stool

Raw lotus root

- *Center burner vacuity:* Lack of appetite (anorexia), nausea, dysphagia (problems or pain when swallowing), diarrhea

Cooked lotus root

- *Blood vacuity:* General fatigue, vertigo (dizziness), recurrent collapses or breakdowns. Recommended especially following childbirth: Lotus root cooked with angelica (*radix angelicae sinensis*) replenishes blood.

Onion

Thermal nature	Warm
Flavor	Acrid and sweet (by lightly braising)
Organ network	Lung, stomach, large intestine
Direction	Upbearing
Effect	Supplements stomach, regulates *qi*, disperses blood stasis, drives out cold, produces perspiration, promotes appetite, loosens *qi* stagnation, and supplements center burner when abdomen is taut and appetite is lacking
Preparation methods	As juice, fried, or dried; onions lose their effect when cooked too long
Contains	High concentration of sulfur-based essential oils (isothiocyanate), many phytonutrients especially the flavonoid quercetin, calcium, iodine, selenium, phosphorus, fluoride, potassium, vitamin B_1, B_2, and C, prostaglandin A, mustard oils

Indications

- Hypertension (high blood pressure), hyperlipidemia (elevated lipoprotein levels in blood plasma), coronary heart disease (Western and Chinese medicine)
- Bronchitis (Western and Chinese medicine)
- *Wind-cold and phlegm disorders:*
  General cold with cold symptoms, bronchitis, sinusitis (loosens phlegm), chest and throat colds

Traditional recipe:
Boil an onion with a teaspoon of honey; apply externally as onion packs or rub on chest.

- *External use for insect bites, swelling, pain:*
  Raw onion or onion juice compress

Contraindications

- *Heat symptoms*
- *General yin vacuity*

Spinach

Thermal nature	Cool
Flavor	Sweet
Organ network	Stomach, liver, large intestine, small intestine
Effect	Clears heat, moistens dryness, promotes the formation of body fluids, supplements blood, supplements liver, supports yin, downbears *qi* (especially of liver and stomach)
Preparation methods	Blanched, as salad or side dish, boiled
Contains	Rich in Vitamin A and C, beta-carotene, folic acid, vitamin B_1, amino acids, phosphorus, oxalic acid, calcium, iron

Indications

- *Heat in stomach:*
  Heartburn, gastritis, gastrointestinal ulcers, thirst, dry mouth, and restlessness
- *Heat symptoms and liver yin vacuity:*
  Headache, dizziness, tinnitus, reddened eyes, restlessness, blurred vision, night blindness, insomnia
- Western indications: Tinnitus, hypertension (blood pressure), following excessive alcohol consumption

Blanch spinach, let cool; season with soy sauce, vinegar, and salt.

- *Heat in blood:*
  Nosebleeds, skin disorders with itching, reddened cutaneous efflorescence

- *Dryness and heat in large intestine:*
  Constipation, anal fistula, hemorrhoids, blood in stool, chronic constipation in elderly people

Contraindications

- *Center burner vacuity* with a tendency to diarrhea

Sweet Potato

Thermal nature	Neutral with a tendency towards warm
Flavor	Sweet
Organ network	Stomach, spleen, kidney
Direction	Upbearing
Phase	Earth
Effect	Supplements center burner and supports formation of *qi* and blood, disperses *qi* stagnation, harmonizes blood, produces fluids, strengthens kidney yin, laxative in its raw form
Contains	Pantothenic acid, vitamin A and C, potassium, magnesium

Indications

- *Stomach qi, spleen qi, or yang vacuity:*
  Diarrhea with "cold symptoms and signs" and weakness; constipation

Contraindications

- *Excessive consumption leads to stagnations in center burner with bloating and distension.*

Tomato

Thermal nature	Cold
Flavor	Sweet and sour
Organ network	Stomach, liver
Direction	Downbearing
Phase	Wood, earth
Effect	Clears heat, enriches yin (especially liver yin), produces fluids and removes dryness, cools and cleans blood, strengthens stomach, promotes liver network activity
Preparation methods	Raw, as juice, boiled, sautéed, or as decoction
Contains	High in vitamin A, B_1, B_2, and C, zinc, cobalt, magnesium, calcium, phosphorus, iron, potassium, essential oils, natural hormones, oxalic acid (caution in case of kidney stones!)

Indications

- *Heat in blood:*
  Nosebleeds, skin disorders with itching, reddened cutaneous efflorescence, sun allergy, seasonal allergies
- *Heat in liver and liver yin vacuity:*
  Headaches, red itching eyes, vertigo (dizziness), tinnitus, night blindness, blurred vision, hypertension (high blood pressure)

Western recommendation:
One to two tomatoes for breakfast.

- *Heat symptoms and yin vacuity of stomach:*
  Thirst, dry throat, lack of appetite, restlessness
- *Heat symptoms and vacuity of body fluids:*
  Restlessness, nervousness

Fresh tomatoes with sugar, mixture of tomatoes and melon juice.

Contraindications

- *Cold and vacuity in center burner*

Constant and excessive consumption of tomatoes, especially during the cold seasons, causes pronounced cooling and weakening of the body. Daily dosage is about one to two tomatoes. Unripe tomatoes and tomatoes with green patches can weaken the kidney network.

Grains and Soy

According to Traditional Chinese Medicine (TCM), grains should make up the main part of one's daily diet. Grains supply the body with strength and endurance, and promote emotional stability, mental calm, and balance (especially wheat).

Grains are mostly sweet and primarily affect the spleen/pancreas and stomach organ network. Their thermal nature is warm, neutral, or cool, depending on the type of grain.

A diet rich in grains ensures a good balance between *qi*, *yin*, and *yang* formation.

With cold symptoms, during the cold season, or when following a primarily vegetarian diet, warming types of grain such as oats or buckwheat should be given preference. In those cases, the thermal energy of grains should be raised by adding warming spices and vegetables like cinnamon, ginger, garlic, raisins, and fennel to the diet.

Soy is listed with grains here (even though it is a legume), because it plays a similar nutritional role in Chinese dietetics.

- To treat **repletion** (strong person, loud, powerful voice, choleric features, extroverted; red tongue, sometimes with thick fur): Wheat, rice, barley.
- To treat **vacuity** (weak person; weak, quiet voice; frequently tired and exhausted; pale, swollen tongue; weak pulse): Oats, rice, spelt, corn, millet.
- To treat **heat** (red tongue, rapid pulse, red face, reddened eyes, nervousness): Wheat, barley, amaranth.
- To treat **cold** (pale, swollen tongue, weak; slow pulse, shivering, aversion to cold, worsening of condition and pain with cold): Oats, rice, corn.
- To treat **dampness** (swelling, edema; chronic phlegm disorders, e.g., frontal sinusitis, bronchitis): Millet, rye, buckwheat, barley.
- To treat **dryness** (dry mouth, lips, and skin; constipation): Wheat, spelt.

Tips for the preparation of grains

In Chinese nutrition, grains are always eaten cooked or as a decoction, **never raw**. Grains can be eaten whole, ground coarsely or finely (preferably freshly ground just before use), or rolled into flakes.

- If at all possible, use organically grown and processed grain. Always rinse grain well before use.
- To shorten the cooking time for grains and to make them more digestible, soak grains for 3–10 hours before cooking. This reduces phytin (phytic acid, inhibits minerals absorption) and makes minerals more available.
- Cook grains in their soaking liquid.
- Soaking is not necessary for millet, buckwheat, rice, or ground corn (polenta).
- To cook grains, use two to two-and-a-half parts of water for each part of grain. For barley, Grünkern (dried, unripe spelt kernels), and especially polenta, three to four parts of water can be used.
- Cook buckwheat, millet, white rice, coarsely, ground grains, or grain flakes for about 20–25 minutes.
- Cook brown rice, spelt kernels, and Grünkern for about 45 minutes.
- Cook wheat, barley, and whole oat kernels for about 1 hour.
- For best results, after cooking, remove pot from heat source and allow grains to sit, covered, for about 30 minutes.
- Salt, herbs, or spices, if desired, should be added to grain dishes after cooking.
- Spices that make grains more digestible: Caraway, fennel, anise, coriander.

Barley

Thermal nature	Cool
Flavor	Salty, sweet
Organ network	Spleen, stomach
Direction	Downbearing
Phase	Earth, water
Effect	Clears heat, moistens dryness, nourishes yin, harmonizes stomach, removes digestive obstructions, detoxifies, increases diuresis (formation and secretion of urine)
Preparation methods	Cooked whole, ground, as flakes, as a decoction, as porridge
Contains	Protein, starch, fat, calcium, vitamin B_1, B_2, and B_6, pantothenic acid, folic acid, calcium, potassium, magnesium, iron, copper, zinc, silicic acid, mucins

Indications

- *Heat symptoms*:
  Agitation, nervousness, insomnia, dryness of mouth

Porridge of freshly ground and cooked barley.

- *Disharmony in center burner (especially stomach):*
  Nausea, vomiting, lack of appetite, abdominal pain due to bloating and food stagnation; supports digestive function

Porridge of freshly ground and cooked barley with slightly warming ingredients, for example raisins and cinnamon.

- *Water accumulation (edema) in body*

Buckwheat

Thermal nature	Varies depending on source, classified mostly as cool, in some sources as warm
Flavor	Sweet
Organ network	Stomach, spleen, large intestine
Phase	Earth
Effect	Downbears *qi*, supplements spleen, loosens hardness, dispels dampness
Preparation methods	Cooked whole or ground as porridge, decoction, or as flower
Contains	Protein, fat, carbohydrates, calcium, phosphorus, iron, potassium, copper, vitamin B_1, B_2, B_3, and E, lecithin, lysine, tryptophane

Indications

- *Stagnation and counterflow stomach qi:*
  Nausea, vomiting, pain, abdominal distention

Contraindications (Depending on Thermal Classification)

- *Warm classification*:
  Excessive consumption of buckwheat can produce heat symptoms and provoke internal upbearing heat syndromes, dizziness, headaches, restlessness, etc.
- *Cool classification*:
  Limit intake for stomach spleen vacuity.

Corn

Thermal nature	Neutral
Flavor	Sweet
Organ network	Kidney, large intestine, stomach
Phase	Earth
Effect	Supplements center burner, kidneys, *qi*, and blood; balances body fluids, harmonizes stomach, strengthens diuresis (production and elimination of urine)
Preparation methods	Boiled, as porridge or decoction
Contains	Protein, fat, starch, iron, phosphorus, vitamin B_1, B_2 B_6, and E, high in unsaturated fatty acids, calcium, potassium, selenium. Suitable for gluten-free diet!

Indications

- *Center burner vacuity:*
  Lack of appetite, indigestion, diarrhea
- *Kidney yin vacuity:*
  Lack of strength, weakness, and sensation of cold in lower extremities, impotence
- *Water accumulation in body:*
  Edema and bloating

Millet

Thermal nature	Neutral to slightly warming (depending on source, some sources classify it as cool)
Flavor	Sweet and salty
Organ network	Stomach, spleen, kidney
Direction	Downbearing
Phase	Earth, water
Effect	Supplements, strengthens, and harmonizes center burner (best grain besides rice for this organ network), strengthens kidneys (very good food during pregnancy), supplements blood and *qi*, dispels dampness, transforms phlegm, downbears counterflow stomach *qi*, diuretic, detoxifying
Preparation methods	Cooked as porridge, decoction, or steamed
Contains	Carbohydrates, protein, starch, fat (high in linoleic acid), calcium, phosphorus, rich in iron, fluoride, magnesium, vitamin B_1 and B_6, lecithin, extremely high in silicic acid

Indications

- *Center burner vacuity:*
  Lack of appetite, general weakness, fatigue, diarrhea

Millet muesli (or porridge) for breakfast, with raisins, nuts, cinnamon, and fruits in season.

- Dampness and phlegm disorders due to spleen vacuity
- Recurrent phlegm disorders (sinusitis, bronchitis), dull feeling of heaviness in head, feeling of heaviness in extremities, nausea, indigestion.
- *Counterflow stomach qi:*
  Acute and chronic nausea, vomiting, morning sickness

- *Stomach and intestinal infections:*
  Following intake of spoiled foods, with acute nausea and diarrhea
- General weakness, lack of strength, and sensation of cold, especially weakness in lower extremities

Oats

Thermal nature	Neutral to warm
Flavor	Sweet
Organ network	Spleen, stomach, kidney
Direction	Upbearing
Phase	Earth, water
Effect	Supplements *qi* and blood, moves *qi*; strengthens nerves, muscles, and sinews; dispels dampness
Preparation methods	Decoction, ground, as porridge, or rolled oats
Contains	Especially valuable protein (contains all essential amino acids), fat, vitamin B_1 and B_2, calcium, iron, manganese, silicon, zinc

Indications

- *General qi, blood, and yang vacuity*
- Exhaustion
- Recovery after extended, chronic, draining illnesses
- General physical lack of strength, especially in pale, weak children and elderly people

Freshly cooked oat porridge daily, or cooked oatmeal with raisins.

Contraindications

- *Use cautiously for heat symptoms*
- Consumed in excess, oats can produce anxiety, nervousness, sleep disturbances ("feeling one's oats").

Rice (White and Brown)

Thermal nature	Neutral
Flavor	Sweet
Organ network	Spleen, stomach, lung
Direction	Upbearing
Phase	Earth
Effect	Supplements *qi* and blood, harmonizes stomach, strengthens spleen, regulates and produces body fluids, relieves diarrhea, diuretic
Preparation methods	Boiled as porridge, steamed, as a decoction
Contains	Carbohydrates, protein, fat; brown rice contains vitamin B_1, B_2, B_3, and E, iron, potassium, all essential amino acids, linoleic acid

Indications

- *Spleen and stomach vacuity:*
  General lack of strength, lack of appetite, nausea, vomiting, morning sickness, diarrhea

Cook short-grain (glutinous) rice in desired amount of water.
Good for infants and children with nausea and vomiting: At first, drink only the boiled rice liquid, later eat the rice, possibly sweetened with honey or licorice.

- *Heat symptoms due to stomach yin vacuity:*
  Thirst, dry mouth, restlessness, insomnia (stabilizes mood swings)

! Rice (along with millet) is recommended for strengthening the stomach and spleen network (short-grain, glutinous rice especially supplements *qi*).
Short-grain (glutinous, sweet, or sticky) rice, with its warming thermal nature, is very suitable for supplementing *qi* and blood.

Basic recipe for congee: (Anglo-Indian: Rice pudding or rice porridge. In Chinese, this dish is called "shi fan" or "water rice"; the main ingredients are rice and water.)

Add one cup of rice (or possibly other grain) to six to ten cups of water. Boil briefly, then simmer on low heat for about four to six hours. Effect: Strengthens *qi* of center burner. This effect can be modified by adding other foods or herbs (see also below).

Examples

Mung bean congee: Cools, lowers fever, especially from summer heat.

Chestnut congee: Strengthens kidney network.

Wheat congee: Strengthens liver *yin*, cools and lowers fever, calms and stabilizes mood.

Rye

Thermal nature	Neutral to cool
Flavor	Bitter
Organ network	Gallbladder, liver, spleen, heart
Direction	Upbearing
Phase	Fire
Effect	Dispels dampness, supports first and foremost the secretion of fluids (diuretic)
Preparation methods	Cooked as decoction, porridge, flour
Contains	Protein, starch, fat, calcium, phosphorus, potassium, zinc, high in lysine, B-vitamins

Indications

- *Phlegm and fluid accumulation*

Spelt

Thermal nature	Neutral to cool
Flavor	Sweet
Organ network	Spleen, stomach, liver
Direction	Downbearing
Phase	Earth
Effect	Similar to wheat (according to TCM), with a slightly more warming thermal nature (less tendency to form dampness and phlegm symptoms). More robust in its cultivation (grown without synthetic agricultural chemicals), valued for its purity
Preparation methods	Ground coarsely, ground as flour, as porridge, flakes, as decoction
Contains	Carbohydrates, protein, starch. fat, lecithin, vitamin B_1 and B_2, zinc, silicic acid, unsaturated fatty acids

Indications

Similar to wheat.

Due to its purity, spelt is the preferred grain in some dietary plans for allergies and skin disorders.

Soybean, Black

Thermal nature	Neutral
Flavor	Sweet
Organ network	Spleen, kidney
Direction	Upbearing
Phase	Earth (water)
Effect	Supplements spleen and kidneys, nourishes kidney yin, moves blood, dispels wind, dispels dampness, detoxifies; strengthens spleen, supplements blood and *qi*, clears heat and drains yang; moistens dryness and supports the excretion of water; used to treat bloating in abdomen, diarrhea, malnutrition in children, severe emaciation, allergies, and skin rashes
Preparation methods	As a decoction, boiled, soaked in alcohol
Contains	Rich in protein, fat and carbohydrates; phosphorus, iron, vitamin B_1 and B_2

Indications

- *Spleen vacuity:*
  Water accumulation, edemas, feeling of oppression, heavy limbs, bloating

Soybean decoction (200 g = about 0.5 lb)

- *Kidney vacuity, especially kidney yin vacuity:*
  Weakness in lower extremities, hearing loss, premature graying of hair, thirst, dry eyes, blurry vision, night sweat, low back pain

Roast black soybeans (200 g = about 0.5 lb) in a dry pan at low temperature until fragrant. Pickle in rice wine for several days, remove beans, and drink 100 mL (about one half cup) of the liquid twice daily.

- *Wind–dampness disorders (damp impediment, shi bi):*
  Rheumatic (arthritis) pain, aching joins, muscle pain that worsens with external dampness and wind

Contraindications

- *Excess weakens spleen and can cause phlegm disorders*

Soybean, Yellow

Thermal nature	Neutral, tendency toward warmth; roasted: hot
Flavor	Sweet
Organ network	Stomach, spleen, large intestine
Direction	Downbearing
Phase	Earth
Effect	Supplements spleen, *qi*, and blood, downbears *qi*, moistens dryness, secretes fluids, detoxifies
Preparation methods	Boiled, powdered, or as decoction
Contains	High in protein, very suitable for treatment of malnutrition. Fats, unsaturated fatty acids, phosphorus, iron, calcium, carotene, vitamin B_1, B_2, and B_{12} folic acid, lysine, lecithin

Indications

- *Weakness of stomach and spleen with qi and blood vacuity:*
  Fatigue, lack of strength, cool extremities, lack of appetite

Warm soymilk

- Water accumulations, edemas, bloating due to spleen weakness
- *Disharmony in large intestine:*
  Acute and chronic indigestion, diarrhea, swell-

ing in abdomen, abdominal distension, especially in toddlers
- After consumption of spoiled foods

Soy beans are high in valuable protein with all essential amino acids and high-quality fatty acids. Soy milk and soy bean products are a preferred treatment for people with skin disorders and allergies, provided they do not have soy allergies or intolerances.

Contraindications

- *Excessive consumption leads to:*
  Qi stagnation in abdomen, abdominal distension and possibly formation of dampness and phlegm

Wheat

Thermal nature	Cool, tendency to cold
Flavor	Sweet
Organ network	Heart, liver, spleen, kidney
Direction	Downbearing
Phase	Earth
Effect	Clears heat, supplements spleen and kidney, nourishes heart yin, builds *qi* and blood when combined with warm foods, relives thirst, diuretic
Preparation methods	Cooked coarsely ground, finely milled, as porridge, or as decoction
Contains	Carbohydrates, protein, starch, fat, lecithin, vitamin B-complex, E, beta-carotene, biotin, folic acid, selenium, natural estrogen

Indications

- *General heat symptoms:*
  Dry mouth, fever, sweating. Well suited for lowering fever in infants and toddlers.

Boil 0.5 L (two cups) water with two tablespoons coarsely ground wheat for 30 minutes, possibly sweeten with licorice; drink while warm.

- *Internal heat conditions with emotional and psychological symptoms:*
  Agitation, anxiety, hysteria, internal restlessness, irritability, insomnia, unstable emotional state, tendency to sadness

Decoction of wheat (220 g or 0.5 lb), Jujube (Chinese dates, 50 g, about 1.5 oz), licorice (18 g, about 0.5 oz); drink warm, twice daily. Wheat is well suited for "inner" emotional stabilization! (Caution: phlegm disorders).

- *Liver heat, for example due to ascending liver yang or liver fire flaming upward:*
  Irritability, disturbed sleep, restlessness, headaches, dizziness, tinnitus, reddened itchy eyes

Freshly ground, cooked wheat porridge (50 g or about 1.5 oz) daily, no meat for one to two weeks, and avoid thermally hot foods, for example acrid spices, alcohol.

- *Liver blood vacuity and blood heat:*
  Itching skin disorders, allergies
- *Menopause:*
  For hot flashes or night sweats

Contraindications

- *Excess wheat or wheat products (pasta) produces dampness and phlegm*

Wheat flour, wheat bran, or wheat germ have significant differences in thermal nature:

Wheat flour	Warm, can cause heat symptoms if eaten in excess
Wheat germ	Cold
Wheat bran	Cool to cold

Wheat supplies the body with strength and endurance.

Spices, Herbs, Sweeteners, Condiments

Sweeteners are warm in thermal nature and sweet in flavor. Spices are usually warm to hot in thermal nature and acrid in flavor.

Due to their warming effect, sweeteners and spices support the center burner and activate the digestive organs. Spices are well suited for "warming" the thermal nature of cool or cold foods. This makes them valuable especially during the cold weather months, or for *qi* or *yang* vacuity of the digestive organs.

Excessive consumption of spices can easily cause heat symptoms, and when occurring over a longer period, can be partially responsible for *yin* vacuity.

- To treat **repletion** (robust person; loud, powerful voice; sensation of heat, hyperactivity, choleric features, extroverted, tongue with thick fur, replete pulse): Avoid hot spices, or use extremely sparingly (caution with garlic, ginger, cinnamon).
- To treat **vacuity** (weak person; weak, quiet voice; shivering, often tired and exhausted, introverted, swollen tongue, weak pulse): Mix fortifying foods with warming spices: garlic, fennel seeds, cinnamon, ginger.
- To treat **heat** (red face, thirst for cold drinks, worsening of condition and pain with heat, red tongue, rapid pulse): Avoid hot and warm spices completely!
- To treat **cold** (shivering, aversion to cold, worsening of condition and pain with cold, pale, swollen tongue; weak, slow pulse): Season foods well, for example with pepper, garlic, ginger, cinnamon, chili, fennel seeds.
- To treat **dampness** (general sensation of heaviness, pathological swelling, edema; chronic phlegm disorders, e.g., frontal sinusitis, bronchitis): Fresh ginger.
- To treat **dryness** (dry mouth, lips, and chapped hands; dry mucous membranes): Avoid hot and warm spices and seasonings completely!

Chili

Thermal nature	Hot
Flavor	Acrid
Organ network	Stomach, spleen, heart
Direction	Upbearing
Phase	Fire
Effect	Dissipates cold, warms center burner, dissolves food stagnation, sweat producing, dries dampness
Preparation methods	Mainly as a seasoning; raw, fried, in soups
Contains	Rich in capsaicin and 2H-capsaicin, essential oils, vitamin C, A, and E, phosphorus, calcium

Indications

- *Wind-cold disorders:*
  Flu, common cold, with aversion to cold; shivering
- *External wind-cold and wetness influences, as well as cold obstructions:*
  Rheumatic disorders or arthrosis worsened by external wind-cold influences
- *Stagnation of cold wetness in center burner:*
  Lack of appetite, fatigue and exhaustion, sensation of heaviness and muscle pain in extremities
- *Cold in stomach and spleen:*
  Decreased appetite, sensation of cold in stomach, diarrhea, nausea, and vomiting

Contraindications

- Generally, all hot chilies and peppers should be used sparingly. They are, however, very well suited as seasoning to supply dishes with a warming effect, if used in focused applications and in moderation.
- *Restraint is advised for patients with general yin vacuity and heat symptoms,* such as dry eyes, ulcers in mouth area, ulcers in digestive tract, and hemorrhoids.

Cinnamon

Thermal nature	Warm to hot
Flavor	Acrid
Organ network	Stomach, spleen, liver, kidney
Direction	Upbearing
Phase	Earth, metal (depending on sources)
Effect	Warms center burner, dissipates cold, moves blood, loosens stagnation; can promote the secretion of digestive juices and alleviate bloating.
Preparation methods	As seasoning or in seasoning mix, powder, decoction, or in pill form
Contains	About 2 % cinnamon oil and 90 % cinnamon aldehyde and resins

Indications

- *Stomach and spleen vacuity:*
  Lack of appetite
- *Cold symptoms, cold in stomach and spleen*
  with sensitivity to cold, abdominal pain, nausea, vomiting, and diarrhea
- *Pain caused by stagnation due to cold or pain due to wind–cold or blood stasis:*
  Abdominal pain (e.g., after childbirth), rheumatic pain (caused by wind–cold and dampness)
- *Wind–cold disorders:*
  Common cold, flu
- *General yang vacuity, spleen yang vacuity, or kidney yang vacuity:*
  Cold extremities, aversion to cold, shivering, cold in lower part of the body, impotence, pain in back and knees, abdominal pain that worsens with cold

Contraindications

- *Heat symptoms due to yin vacuity*
- Restricted use during pregnancy

Coriander

Green leaves, stems, roots, and dried seeds of plant

Thermal nature	Warm
Flavor	Acrid
Organ network	Lung, spleen
Direction	Upbearing
Phase	Metal
Effect	Well suited for warming foods; dissipates cold, produces perspiration, balances *qi*, disperses blood stasis, loosens digestive obstruction, reverses counterflow *qi*
Preparation methods	Use leaves, stems, roots, or dried seeds in soups; as salad, or as a seasoning; should not be cooked too long to retain warming effect
Contains	Essential oils, bioflavonoids, protein, vitamin C, and calcium

Indications

- *Cold and disharmony in stomach and spleen*:
  Lack of appetite, nausea, indigestion, digestive stagnation due to cold influences in abdomen

Add coriander as a seasoning to dishes.

- *Wind–cold disorders:*
  Colds, flu with aversion to cold, chills, low-grade fever, little sweat

Decoction of green onions, coriander seeds, and ginger.

Contraindications

- *Use with caution in cases of:*
  General *qi* vacuity or foul-smelling perspiration

Ginger, Fresh or Dried

Thermal nature	Warm (dried ginger is warmer)
Flavor	Acrid (dried ginger is more acrid)
Organ network	Lung, stomach, spleen
Direction	Upbearing
Phase	Metal
Effect	Strengthens center burner, controls nausea, frees surface from pathogenic wind–cold factors (supports stomach *qi* in the Greater Yang layer (tai yang), sweat-producing, relieves retching, transforms phlegm, supplements lung, relieves cough and detoxifies; stimulates blood circulation, increases appetite, and promotes secretion of digestive juices
Preparation method	Fresh ginger (purple ginger is milder and is often eaten as a vegetable); dried ginger flakes, chips, or powder; as juice or decoction
Contains	High in essential oils, starch and amino acids, amaroids (bitters), gingereol = cardio tonic agent (activates Ca2+-pumping ATPase in skeletal and cardiac sarcoplasmic reticulum)

Dried ginger (powder, chips, or candied) is classified as hotter than fresh ginger in thermal nature.

Indications

- *Stomach and spleen vacuity, disharmony of stomach qi (wei qi bu he), stomach qi upbearing counterflow (wei qi shang ni):*
  Nausea and vomiting

Chewing a small slice of fresh or crystallized (candied) ginger is a great remedy for motion sickness and morning sickness.

- *Cold, flu caused by wind–cold:*
  Chills, aversion to cold, arthritis/joint pain, headaches, stuffed up nose

Decoction of fresh ginger and green onions:
Simmer thumb-sized pieces of ginger and green onions in 0.5 L (two cups) of water for 10 minutes; drink warm decoction immediately at the first sign of a cold .

- *Cold in lung or cold phlegm:*
  Cough, shortness of breath, clear, white phlegm

Decoction of fresh ginger with malt sugar (or raw cane sugar or molasses): Combine about 50 g (1.5 oz) of ginger and 30 g (one to two tablespoons) of malt sugar into a decoction and drink warm.

- *Indigestion:*
  Vomiting and diarrhea after consumption of spoiled foods

Freshly grated ginger, possibly as a tea.

- *General cold symptoms:*
  Cold hands and feet, rheumatism (arthritis) that worsens with wind–cold

Contraindications

- *General yin vacuity and heat signs*
- High blood pressure

Prolonged consumption of larger amounts of ginger should be avoided. Excess can provoke heat phlegm disorders.

Garlic

Thermal nature	Cooked: warm Raw: hot
Flavor	Raw: acrid Gently cooked: sweet–acrid
Organ network	Lung, stomach, spleen
Direction	Upbearing
Phase	Earth
Effect	Warms center burner, strengthens stomach, moves *qi*, disperses blood stasis and *qi* stagnation in abdomen, dispels cold, detoxifies, antiparasitic, relieves cough
Preparation methods	Raw, gently braised (on low heat), as a juice or decoction
Contains	High in essential oils, mainly allicin (antibiotic effect), protein, calcium, vitamin B_1 and C, carotene

Raw garlic is significantly more acrid and is classified as thermally hot, while gently braised garlic develops a sweet flavor and is classified as having a warm/hot thermal nature.

Indications

- Cold symptoms and digestive obstructions in center burner:
  Pain in abdomen and solar plexus (epigastric) region

Garlic cloves pickled in vinegar, about half a clove once daily

- *Nausea, vomiting, diarrhea, or dysentery,* also in connection with intake of contaminated food

Garlic raw or braised

- *Intense watery diarrhea*

Garlic syrup:
Chop one clove of garlic, mix with one tablespoon of lemon juice and one tablespoon of honey. Take this mixture three to five times a day.

- *Cold, cough, or whooping-cough, chronic and acute bronchitis*

Decoction of garlic, ginger, and sugar.

- *Parasite infestation,* especially hookworms and pinworms (enterobiasis, oxyuriasis)

10–15 g (0.5 oz) steamed garlic with sunflower seeds.

- Prophylaxis for flu, hypertension (high blood pressure) and hyperlipidemia

Contraindications

- *Heat symptoms*
- *General yin vacuity*
- Thrush (aphtha)

In Western medicine, the regular intake of garlic shows a positive effect on stomach peristalsis and secretion. Garlic glycosides can lower blood pressure and can decrease blood lipids and thus may be good prevention for arteriosclerosis. Garlic also has a known antibacterial and antiparasitic effect.

Mushrooms

Thermal nature	Cool to cold
Flavor	Sweet
Organ network	Stomach, spleen, lung
Direction	Downbearing
Phase	Earth
Effect	Support center burner, balance *qi*, moisten dryness, transform phlegm
Preparation methods	Boiled, steamed, or powdered
Contains	Protein, fat, calcium, potassium, phosphorus, iron, zinc, magnesium, vitamins A, B_1, B_2, C, E, and K, essential amino acids, dietary fiber, high purine concentration (contraindicated for people suffering from gout)

Indications

- *Spleen and stomach qi vacuity*:
  Lack of appetite, fatigue, nausea, vomiting, reduced milk flow

Cooked mushrooms with chicken (or pork)

- *Lung yin vacuity*:
  Shortness of breath, dry cough with viscous phlegm

Contraindications

- Excessive consumption can lead to possible heavy-metal exposure

Pepper (Seasoning)

Thermal nature	Hot
Flavor	Acrid
Organ network	Stomach, spleen, large intestine, lung
Direction	Upbearing
Phase	Metal
Effect	Warms center burner, dissipates cold, regulates *qi*, disperses blood stasis, reduces counterflow *qi*, eliminates phlegm, relieves pain, produces sweat, dispels wind–cold, disperses *qi* stagnation and blood stasis. In small amounts, pepper promotes secretion of digestive juices, increases appetite, and alleviates bloating.
Preparation methods	As a seasoning, decoction, powder, or pill
Contains	Essential oils, piperine, piperonal, calcium, iron

Indications

- *General spleen and stomach vacuity:*
  Lack of appetite, indigestion, bloating

Increase use of pepper as a seasoning.

- *Cold disorders of stomach and spleen:*
  Sensation of cold and pain in abdomen. Pain that worsens with cold.

Decoction of pepper and ginger: Simmer a pinch of freshly ground pepper and 30 g (1 oz) fresh ginger in water for 10 minutes. Drink while warm.

- *Cold phlegm disorders:*
  Clear or white sputum

- *Wind–cold disorders:*
  Cold with cough, hoarseness, cold limbs. Rheumatoid arthritis due to wind–cold influences

Contraindications

- *Heat symptoms due to general yin vacuity:*
  Excessive consumption of pepper damages body fluids (dehydrates)

Salt

Thermal nature	Cold
Flavor	Salty
Organ network	Stomach, kidney, small intestine, and large intestine
Direction	Downbearing
Phase	Water
Effect	Clears heat, cools blood, moistens dryness, downbears *qi*, strengthens kidneys, loosens phlegm
Preparation methods	As seasoning, dissolved in warm or hot water

Indications

- *Kidney yin and yang vacuity*:
  Supplements the kidney organ network when taken in moderation
- *Fire flaming upward due to yin vacuity:*
  Dizziness, headaches, red eyes, mouth and tongue ulcers, bleeding gums, constipation, hoarseness and sore throat

Half a teaspoon of salt dissolved in warm water, taken before meals.

- *Phlegm accumulation or hardness in body*

Contraindications

- Shortness of breath
- Edema
- Diabetes mellitus
- High blood pressure

Seaweed (General)

Thermal nature	Cold
Flavor	Salty
Organ network	Liver, lung, kidneys
Direction	Downbearing
Phase	Water
Effect	Clears heat, moistens dryness, transforms phlegm, softens hardness, enriches yin, diuretic
Preparation methods	Fresh or dried, boiled, as a soup ingredient, as a decoction, as salad, as pill or powder
Contains	41 minerals and trace elements, unsurpassed source of iodine, vitamin A, B_1, B_6, B_{12}, C, D, E, and K

Indications

- *Heat and phlegm in lung*, bronciectasis or cough with viscous yellow phlegm
- *Following excessive alcohol consumption with heat symptoms*
- *Edema*

Contraindications

- Seaweed should not be consumed in excess (iodine!)

Soy Sauce

Thermal nature	Cold
Flavor	Salty and sweet
Organ network	Spleen, stomach, kidney
Direction	Downbearing
Phase	Water
Effect	Clears heat, harmonizes center burner, detoxifies
Contains	Protein, fat, glucose, calcium, phosphorus, vitamin B_1 and B_2, niacin, iron

Indications

- *Disharmony of stomach qi:* Lack of appetite, nausea
- *Heat symptoms:* Agitation, nervousness
- *Symptoms of stomach poisoning* due to spoiled foods such as meat and fish

Contraindications

- Formation of phlegm possible with excessive consumption

Sweeteners: Brown or Whole Cane Sugar

Made from the pressed juice of sugar cane. Preferably raw, unrefined, and made with whole sugar cane, without removal of molasses (e.g., Rapadura).

Thermal nature	Warm
Flavor	Sweet
Organ network	Spleen, stomach, liver
Direction	Upbearing
Phase	Earth
Effect	Supplements center burner, supplements *qi*, disperses blood stasis, calms liver, moves and harmonizes blood, relieves spasms and acute pain
Preparation methods	Dissolved in warm liquids, in alcoholic beverages, as decoction
Contains	Sucrose, calcium, vitamin B_2, iron

Indications

- *Stomach and spleen vacuity:* Abdominal pain, for example with blood stasis, nausea, and vomiting

Decoction of brown sugar (100 g or about 2.5 oz), fresh ginger (200 g or about 5 oz), and dried tangerine peels.

- *Blood stasis caused by cold:* Painful menstruation, persisting and congesting lochia (postnatal discharge) following childbirth

Contraindications

- *Dampness and phlegm disorders*
- *Damp–heat*
- Dental cavities (caries)

Sweeteners: Honey

Thermal nature	Neutral
Flavor	Sweet
Organ network	Spleen, lung, large intestine
Direction	Upbearing
Phase	Earth
Effect	Supplements center burner, moistens dryness, moistens lung, relieves cough, relieves pain, moistens large intestine, detoxifies
Preparation methods	Raw, as a seasoning in cooking, dissolved in warm water
Contains	About 70 % fructose and glucose, also protein, citric acid, pectin; small amounts of vitamin A, B_1, B_2, B_6, C, and D, magnesium, calcium, potassium, sodium, phosphorus, iron, copper, manganese

Indications

- *Stomach and spleen vacuity:*
  Lack of appetite, fatigue, lack of strength, shortness of breath, diarrhea with abdominal pain
- *Dryness of lung:*
  Dry cough with little sputum or with viscous phlegm, hoarseness, dry throat, chronic hacking and exhaustion cough

Steamed pear with honey

- *Dryness in large intestine with vacuity of body fluids due to heat:*
  Constipation, especially constipation in elderly people

Mix honey with roasted black sesame; grind into porridge; dissolve in warm water and drink.

- *Stomach heat:*
  Gastritis, stomach and duodenal ulcers
- *External application*:
  Chapped and dry lips, ulcers in mouth or lips, burns or frostbites

Contraindications

- *Dampness and phlegm disorders*
- *Stagnation in center burner*
- Diarrhea

Sweeteners: Malt Sugar–Maltose–Malt Syrup

Formed by enzymes or acid hydrolysis from starch (grains or tubers). A natural sweetener usually made from grain (e.g., ground corn and sprouted barley). Found in health-food stores, malt syrup has an earthy, full-bodied flavor and is 75–80 % as sweet as honey. Malt syrup is also referred to as malt extract.

Thermal nature	Warm
Flavor	Sweet
Organ network	Spleen, stomach, lung
Direction	Upbearing
Phase	Earth
Effect	Warms and supplements center burner, moistens the lung, cough-relieving, removes dryness, relieves cramps and acute pain conditions, creates body fluids, detoxifies
Preparation methods	Syrup or powder, dissolve in water, as powder or decoction
Contains	Maltose, vitamin B, iron

Indications

- *Stomach and spleen vacuity*:
  General fatigue, lack of appetite, lack of strength, diarrhea
- *Dryness and lung vacuity:*
  Throat pain, hoarseness, cough with little sputum, shortness of breath

Steam white radish (500 g or about 1 lb) mixed with malt sugar (20 g or about one tablespoon), until sugar has melted (or use malt syrup); eat while warm.

Contraindications

- *Dampness*
- *Moist–heat*
- Bloating in abdomen with tendency to nausea and vomiting

Sweeteners: White Sugar

Made by repeatedly refining and processing the juice of sugar cane, sugar beets, sorghum, or sugar maples.

Thermal nature	Warm to neutral
Flavor	Sweet
Organ network	Stomach, spleen, lung
Direction	Upbearing
Phase	Earth
Effect	Supplements center burner, moistens lung, creates body fluids, alleviates acute pain
Preparation methods	Dissolved in water
Contains	Sucrose

Indications

- *Dryness in lung:*
  Dry cough, hoarseness
- *Stomach yin vacuity:*
  Thirst, dry throat
- *Stomach and spleen vacuity:*
  Painful solar plexus (epigastric) area, or after alcohol excess

Dissolve 30 g (1 oz) of sugar in water.

Contraindications

- *Quickly leads to dampness and phlegm conditions, wet heat*
- *Weakens the kidney network (caries, bones)*

Vinegar

Thermal nature	Warm
Flavor	Sour and bitter
Organ network	Stomach, liver
Direction	Upbearing
Phase	Wood
Effect	Stops bleeding (hemostatic), disperses blood and *qi* stagnation, detoxifies, promotes digestion
Preparation methods	As a seasoning, diluted in water, as decoction
Contains	Acetic acid, acetal, oxalic acid, acetaldehyde, minerals, acids, alcohols of higher quality

Indications

- *Blood stasis:*
  Pain in abdomen, palpable hardness in abdomen

Healing herbs brewed with vinegar.

- *Qi and blood stasis:*
  Digestive obstruction caused by too much fatty, oily food, meat, and fish
- *Bleeding:*
  Nosebleeds, bloody stool, bloody sputum

> **Tip:** Vinegar (as well as celery) is one of the few foods that can treat *qi* and blood stasis. Look for good quality!

Contraindications

- *Stagnation in center burner caused by dampness*

Fruit

Fruits have a sweet, sour, and occasionally bitter flavor. Their thermal nature is primarily cool to cold; for some types of fruit, it is neutral and warm. Fruit should be eaten primarily during the warm and hot seasons since it cools heat conditions, replenishes body fluids, and moistens dryness. In TCM, fruit is a nutritional complement to grains and supports the formation and preservation of body fluids. During the cold season, highly cooling fruit such as bananas, oranges, and lemons should be avoided to prevent developing cold in the body.

- To treat **repletion** (robust person, loud powerful voice, sensation of heat, hyperactivity, choleric features, extroverted, tongue with thick fur, replete pulse): Apple, citrus fruit, pineapple, tangerine.
- To treat **vacuity** (weak person, weak quiet voice, shivering, often tired and exhausted, introverted, swollen tongue, weak pulse): Cherries, red grapes.
- To treat **heat** (red face, thirst for cold drinks, worsening of condition and pain due to heat, red tongue, rapid pulse): Citrus fruit, kiwi, watermelon, pineapple, apple.
- To treat **dryness** (dry mouth and lips, chapped hands, dry mucous membranes): Pear, banana, kiwi.

Apple

Thermal nature	Sweet
Flavor	Sweet and sour
Organ network	Stomach, spleen, lung
Direction	Downbearing
Phase	Earth/wood
Effect	Clears heat, relieves agitation, alleviates summer heat, creates body fluids, moistens the lung, relieves diarrhea, stimulates appetite
Preparation methods	Raw, cooked, as juice, decoction, syrup, dried, as powder
Contains	Calcium, potassium, iron, sodium, phosphorus, sulfur, vitamin A, B_1, B_2, and C, niacin, flavones, malic acid, citric acid, pectin, tannin

Indications

- *Heat symptoms:*
  Restlessness, thirst, or following excessive alcohol consumption

Raw apples

- *Yin vacuity:*
  Lack of appetite, indigestion

Shredded apple, preferably slightly heated or as a compote

Apricot

Thermal nature	Neutral to warm
Flavor	Sweet and sour
Organ network	Stomach, lung
Phase	Earth, wood
Effect	Creates body fluids, moistens lung, quenches thirst and relieves cough
Preparation methods	Raw, dried, as a decoction or syrup
Contains	Very high in minerals and trace elements, iron, potassium and beta-carotene; some silicic acid

Tip: **Due to their high iron content and warming effect, apricots are recommended during pregnancy.**

Indications

- *Stomach yin vacuity:*
  Thirst, dry mouth

Eat fresh apricots.

- *Heat and lung dryness with upbearing qi:*
  Cough, shortness of breath, dry throat, dry cough with viscous phlegm, asthma symptoms

Raw apricots or syrup from apricots preserved in honey.

Contraindications

- *Heat symptoms*
- Diarrhea

! Excessive consumption can damage teeth, especially in children.

Banana

Thermal nature	Cold
Flavor	Sweet
Organ network	Stomach, large intestine
Direction	Downbearing
Phase	Earth
Effect	Clears heat, enriches yin, moistens and detoxifies intestines, creates body fluids, moistens stomach
Preparation methods	Raw or steamed
Contains	10 different vitamins and 18 (!) minerals and trace elements, especially potassium, magnesium, calcium, high in pantothenic acid and folic acid; contains serotonin (good mood hormone!)

Indications

- *Heat disorders that damage yin, especially stomach yin:*
  Thirst, dry throat, restlessness, chronic dry cough, dry stools

Raw bananas

- *Dryness in small and large intestine:*
  Constipation, bleeding hemorrhoids

Raw bananas

Contraindications

- *Cold and vacuity symptoms in center burner*
- Phlegm disorders

Cherry

Thermal nature	Warm
Flavor	Sweet
Organ network	Stomach, spleen (liver and kidney)
Direction	Upbearing
Phase	Earth
Effect	Supplements the center burner, *qi*, and blood; supplements and moistens liver and spleen, disperses blood stasis, dissipates cold, dispels wind–dampness
Preparation methods	Raw, as decoction, syrup, or preserved in alcohol
Contains	Beta-carotene, vitamin B_1, B_2, B_3, and C potassium, calcium, iron, fruit acids, fructose

Indications

- *Spleen and stomach vacuity, stomach yin vacuity:*
  Exhaustion, lack of appetite, fatigue, dryness of skin and mouth

Cherry decoction

- *Liver and kidney vacuity:*
  Weakness and pain in knees and hips, weakness and numbness in limbs

Medicinal cherry wine:
Cover 250 g (about 0.5 lb) of cherries for half a day with 0.5 L (two cups) clear brandy; drink half a cup daily.

- *Wind–dampness:*
  Arthritis pain in lower half of body, rheumatism, gout, arthritis

Cherry juice or medicinal cherry wine

- *Liver and kidney vacuity or stagnation* combined with weak muscles, sinews and bones; weakness of limbs and restricted joint mobility

- *Blood vacuity:*
  Vertigo (dizziness), forgetfulness, heart palpitations, insomnia, restlessness, anemia during pregnancy

Medicinal wine made from cherries and longans

- *Cold disorders*, especially in patients with a tendency to feel cold

Contraindications

- *Exercise restraint with strong heat symptoms*

Grapefruit, Pomelo

Thermal nature	Cool to cold (peel: warm)
Flavor	Sweet and sour (peel: sweet and bitter)
Organ network	Stomach, lung (peel: stomach–kidney–gallbladder)
Direction	Downbearing
Phase	Earth
Effect	Flesh: creates body fluids, relieves thirst Peel: transforms phlegm, downbears *qi* and disperses digestive obstructions
Contains	Vitamin C, beta-carotene, potassium, calcium, amaroids (bitters)

Indications

- *Stomach yin vacuity:*
  Restlessness, thirst, following excessive alcohol consumption

Eat raw grapefruit flesh

- *Stomach qi upbearing counterflow:*
  Nausea, vomiting, stomach aches, diarrhea, digestive obstruction

Simmer whole fruit, including peel, add sugar or honey to taste.
Use only untreated fruit, preferably from organic agriculture.

- *Phlegm disorder, especially of the lung:*
  Bronchitis with viscous, yellow phlegm

Grapefruit with honey for phlegm disorder

Grapes

Thermal nature	Neutral
Flavor	Sweet and sour
Organ network	Spleen, lung, kidneys (liver)
Direction	Downbearing and upbearing
Phase	Wood and earth
Effect	Supplements kidneys and liver, supplements *qi*, promotes blood formation, creates body fluids, strengthens muscles, sinews, and bones; diuretic
Preparation methods	Raw, as juice, decoction, or preserved in alcohol
Contains	Especially rich in glucose, various fruit acids, the highest potassium content in fruit, iron, copper, bioflavonoids

Note: Raisins (dried grapes) have a higher carbohydrate content and more iron and calcium than fresh grapes.

Indications

- *General liver and kidney vacuity:*
  Weakness and pain in knees and hips, rheumatic symptoms with joint pain, caused by wind–dampness and *qi* stagnation
- Weakness and pain in spine, frailty

Medicinal wine made from grapes and ginseng:
Soak equal amounts of fresh grapes (about 10 grapes) and ginseng root in 100 mL (half a cup) brandy for two to four days. Drink 20 mL (about two tablespoons) daily.

- *Stomach and kidney yin vacuity:*
  Dry mouth, thirst, agitation, lack of appetite with a deficiency in body fluids

Syrup made from grapes and honey

- *Qi and blood vacuity:*
  Agitation, dizziness, forgetfulness, night sweat, heart palpitations

Decoction or syrup from raisins

Dried grapes (raisins) have a stronger strengthening effect on the kidney and liver and form *qi* and blood, while fresh grapes primarily create body fluids.

Kiwi

Thermal nature	Cold
Flavor	Sweet and sour
Organ network	Stomach, gallbladder (kidney)
Direction	Downbearing
Phase	Earth, wood
Effect	Clears heat, creates body fluids, harmonizes stomach, downbears upbearing stomach *qi*, diuretic
Contains	Rich in vitamin C (about twice as much as in citrus fruit), some iron, magnesium, proteopeptic enzyme actinidine

Kiwis are believed to lower the carcinogenic effect of nitrosamines in the body, as well as lowering cholesterol and glycerides.

Indications

- *Heat symptoms:*
  Thirst and dryness of the mouth

Raw or as a decoction; peel two to three kiwi and cut into small pieces, add honey and possibly some water and simmer gently

- Diabetes, restlessness

See above

- *Disharmony in stomach and stomach qi upbearing counterflow:*
  Nausea, decreased appetite

Juice mixture of kiwi and ginger: Mix freshly squeezed juice of three kiwis and about one tablespoon juice of freshly squeezed ginger (squeezed separately); drink juice in three portions throughout the day.

- Micturition (urination) difficulties with *heat and dampness symptoms*:
  Painful, sparse micturition, secretion of concrements (stones or crystals in urinary tract)

Raw or as a juice

Contraindications

- *Cold disturbances of stomach and spleen*

Lemon

Thermal nature	Cool to cold
Flavor	Sour
Organ network	Stomach, liver, lung
Direction	Contracting (astringent), downbearing
Phase	Wood
Effect	Clears heat, quenches thirst, dispels summer heat, creates body fluids, harmonizes stomach, and calms the fetus, transforms phlegm, relieves cough
Preparation methods	Raw, as juice, salted or sweetened or as decoction; salted lemon loosens phlegm
Contains	High in vitamin C, also citric acid, malic acid, saccharide, vitamin B_1 and B_2, calcium, phosphorus, potassium

Indications

- *Heat or summer heat symptoms or heat in stomach:*
  Thirst, agitation, sweating, nervousness

Drink lemon juice mixed with sugar cane, raw cane sugar, or Rapadura;

Freshly squeezed lemon juice (one to two lemons daily) for scratchy and burning throat (external wind–heat); gargle.

- *Stomach qi upbearing counterflow*:
  Nausea, vomiting, belching, lack of appetite

Salted lemon

- *Heat phlegm disorders:*
  Bronchitis, sinusitis
- *Liver qi stagnation:*
  Irritability, mood swings, intercostal neuralgia, constipation, inner tension, temporal headache, menopausal symptoms

Decoction of lemon peels together with grapefruit peels moves and regulates liver qi. Please use only peel from organic lemons or grapefruit to prevent possible exposure to agricultural chemicals.

Contraindications

- Stomach hyperacidity and gastric ulcers

Lemons are four to six times more acidic than oranges.

Orange

Thermal nature	Cool to cold
Flavor	Sweet and sour
Organ network	Stomach, gallbladder
Direction	Downbearing
Phase	Wood
Effect	Cools, creates body fluids, thirst-quenching, downbears *qi*
Preparation method	Raw, as juice or decoction
Contains	Vitamin C, beta-carotene, extremely high in bioflavonoids, potassium, magnesium, calcium, iron, saccharide, citric acid

Indications

- *Stomach yin vacuity and heat in stomach:*
  Thirst, restlessness, after excessive consumption of alcohol

Fresh oranges or orange juice with honey

- *Rebellious stomach qi due to heat:*
  Nausea, vomiting

Simmer one to two oranges (peeled) and mix with honey

- *Heat accumulation in lower burner* with painful urination, fever, summer heat
- Sweat-producing physical exertion

Contraindications

- *General cold syndrome:*
  Especially with *qi* vacuity or *yang* vacuity of stomach and spleen
- *Cold disorders of lung*
- *High phlegm accumulation*

Peach

Thermal nature	Warm to hot
Flavor	Sweet–sour
Organ network	Stomach, large intestine (liver)
Direction	Downbearing, upbearing (not certain)
Phase	Earth
Effect	Creates body fluids, moistens intestines, moves blood, dissolves blood stasis, can soften hardness
Preparation methods	Raw, steamed, or dried
Contains	Ripe peaches are rich in vitamins A, B, and C beta-carotene; also bioflavonoids, potassium, calcium, magnesium, iron, zinc. Very favorable potassium–sodium ratio: invigorates kidneys

Indications

- *Stomach yin vacuity:*
  Thirst, dry throat, constipation
- *Heat and dryness in large intestine:*
  Constipation, especially chronic constipation in elderly people

Eat fruit raw or steamed

- *Blood stasis:*
  Painful menstruation

Contraindications

- *Heat symptoms:*
  Especially heat-related skin disorders, *heat in blood*

Pear

Thermal nature	Cool
Flavor	Sweet
Organ network	Lung, stomach
Direction	Downbearing
Phase	Wood, earth
Effect	Clears heat, moistens dryness, creates body fluids, transforms phlegm
Contains	Beta-carotene, vitamin B_1, B_2, B_3 (niacin), and B_6, folic acid, vitamin C, especially rich in potassium; also magnesium, calcium, iron, phosphorus, fruit acids, tannin, hormone-like substances

Indications

- *Heat syndrome with fluid vacuity:*
  Restlessness, sleeplessness, dry mouth
- Heat symptoms in lung and small intestine:
  Trouble swallowing, sore throat

Pure pear juice

- Irritated, hoarse vocal chords, loss of voice, dysphagia, dry cough

Pure pear juice

- Dry, compact stool; constipation

One to two glasses of pure pear juice, at room temperature, taken before noon

- *Heat phlegm disorders of lung:*
  Bronchitis, sinusitis with viscous yellow phlegm

Mixture of pear juice (or concentrated pear syrup)and lemon juice, 200–700 g (one to three cups) daily; loosens and transforms phlegm.

- *Wind-heat symptoms in heart:*
  Thirst, mental restlessness, nervousness, and anxiety

Pineapple

Thermal nature	Neutral to cool
Flavor	Sweet and sour
Organ network	Stomach, gallbladder
Direction	Upbearing
Phase	Earth
Effect	Disperses summer heat, creates body fluids, thirst-quenching, diuretic, promotes digestion
Preparation methods	Raw, as juice or decoction
Contains	High water content, few calories, potassium, calcium, phosphorus, iron, copper, zinc, valuable fruit acids, vitamin C, bromelain enzyme (promotes digestion of protein!)

Indications

- *Heat symptoms and stomach yin vacuity:*
  Thirst, dry mouth, nausea, lack of appetite, restlessness

Fresh pineapple or pineapple juice

- Micturition (urination) problems, dampness in body, fever

Contraindications

- Skin ulcers and eczema

! Unripe, sour pineapples can damage teeth!

Plum

Thermal nature	Neutral to warm
Flavor	Sweet and sour
Organ network	Liver, kidney, stomach
Direction	Upbearing and downbearing
Phase	Earth, wood, water
Effect	Clears liver heat, disperses *qi* stagnation and blood stasis, creates body fluids, diuretic
Preparation methods	Raw, dried, as a juice, or preserved in alcohol
Contains	Excellent potassium–sodium ratio, rich in iron, ideal calcium/phosphorus content, vitamin B_1, B_2, and C, minimal protein and fat

Indications

- *Liver stagnation and heat in liver:*
  Restlessness, irritability, constipation, tendency to outbursts of rage; subfebrile (lower than normal) body temperature in the afternoon, night sweat

Drink fresh plum juice, possibly sweetened with honey

- *Stomach yin vacuity:*
  Thirst, dry mouth

Raw plums or plum juice

- *Formation of ascites* (abdominal fluids) due to liver disorders

Contraindications

Excess

- *Weakens stomach and spleen*
- Decreases appetite
- Leads to diarrhea
- Possibly develops phlegm

Watermelon

Thermal nature	Cold
Flavor	Sweet
Organ network	Stomach, heart, bladder
Direction	Downbearing
Phase	Earth
Effect	Clears heat, relieves summer heat, quenches thirst, relieves agitation, diuretic
Preparation methods	Raw, as a juice, decoction, or syrup
Contains	95% water, high in potassium, calcium, phosphorus, magnesium, iron, zinc, nickel, vitamin A and C, as well as sugar and amaroids

Indications

- Heat and summer heat symptoms, body fluids injured by heat:
  Thirst, restlessness, sweating. During summer heat: Sweating, headaches, dry lips

Eat about 500 g (1 lb) of watermelon fresh or as juice (two cups), possibly mixed with tomato juice.

- *Heat or heart fire flaming upward:*
  Thirst, mouth or tongue ulcers, mental restlessness, disturbed sleep (especially during summer), dark urine, heart palpitations
- *Moist–heat in lower burner:*
  Sparse, dark urine, painful urination

Contraindications

- *Vacuity and cold symptoms in spleen and stomach*
- *General accumulation of moisture*

Meat and Poultry

Most types of meat are warm to hot in thermal nature and are excellent for supplementing *qi* and *yang*. Meat should be eaten primarily during the cold seasons. Meat intensifies body energy and provides the body with a degree of "aggressiveness." It is very suitable for quickly replenishing energy deficits (following heavy physical exertion, after childbirth, during recovery). Excess consumption of meat pollutes the body with toxins and promotes phlegm disorders.

- To treat **repletion** (strong person, loud powerful voice, choleric features, extroverted, red tongue, possibly thick fur): Avoid meat, no meat for four to six weeks; increase grains, fruit, and vegetables.
- To treat **vacuity** (weak person, weak, quiet voice, often tired and exhausted, pale, swollen tongue, weak pulse): Beef, chicken, pork, venison.
- To treat **heat** (red tongue, rapid pulse, red face, reddened eyes, nervousness): No meat for four to six weeks; increase grains, fruit, and vegetables.
- To treat **cold** (pale, swollen tongue, weak, slow pulse, shivering, aversion to cold, cold worsens condition and pain): Above all venison, lamb, game; also chicken, beef.
- To treat **dampness** (swellings, edema, chronic phlegm disorders [e.g., frontal sinusitis, bronchitis]): Avoid meat, no meat for four to six weeks; increase drying grains.
- To treat **dryness** (dry mouth, lips and skin; constipation): Pork, increase grains, fruit and vegetables.

Beef

Thermal nature	Warm, neutral
Flavor	Sweet
Organ network	Spleen, stomach, in part also kidney
Direction	Upbearing
Phase	Earth
Effect	Supplements *qi* and blood, supplements stomach and spleen, strengthens yang, strengthens sinews, muscles and bones
Preparation methods	Boiled, steamed, fried/roasted, or in soup
Contains	Protein, fat, vitamin B_1 and B_2, calcium, phosphorus, iron

Indications

- *Qi and blood vacuity:*
  Lack of strength, weakness in knees and legs, spontaneous sweating, emaciation, especially weakness caused by profuse bleeding after pregnancy or strong menstrual blood losses

Beef stock or beef stew combined with carrots, celery, spinach, mangold chard; very good for supplementing blood, especially during and after pregnancy

- *Stomach and spleen vacuity:*
  Lack of appetite, general weakness, lack of strength, bloating, diarrhea

Beef stock or beef stew combined with carrots, leeks, and onions

Contraindications

- *Meat excess can cause moist–heat symptoms*
- *Exercise restraint also with heat in blood:*
  Skin efflorescence with raised, itching red skin patches, skin ulcers

Beef Liver

Preferably from organically raised or grass-fed animals

Thermal nature	Neutral
Flavor	Sweet
Organ network	Spleen, liver
Direction	Upbearing
Phase	Earth
Effect	Supplements liver network, *qi*, and blood
Preparation methods	Fried or boiled

Indications

- *Especially for blood vacuity:*
  Pale dull complexion, poor concentration, numbness, fatigue, heart palpitations, lack of strength
- *Liver blood vacuity:*
  Night blindness, hypomenorrhea (scant, brief menstruation) or amenorrhea (lack of menstruation), blurred vision, dizziness, insomnia

Beef liver combined with green vegetables and green salads, apple

Chicken

Thermal nature	Warm
Flavor	Sweet
Organ network	Stomach, spleen
Direction	Upbearing
Phase	Earth
Effect	Supports and warms center burner, supplements *qi* and blood, enriches yang, supports ying, supplements bone marrow, enriches kidney yin and yang
Preparation methods	Boiled, steamed, fried/roasted, deep-fried, grilled, or in soup
Contains	Protein, low in fat with high-quality unsaturated fatty acids, calcium, phosphorus, iron

Indications

- *Qi vacuity:*
  Pale face, fatigue, quiet voice, sweating during the day, lack of strength, easily exhausted
- *Blood vacuity (generally associated with qi vacuity):*
  Dull, pale complexion; difficulty concentrating, numbness, muscle weakness, heart palpitations, amenorrhea (lack of menstruation) or hypomenorrhea (scant menstruation), general weakness, emotional instability, depression
- *Qi and blood vacuity following childbirth:*
  Lack of strength, postnatal depression, heart palpitations, dizziness, lack of milk flow after giving birth

Recipe for supplementing qi and blood during pregnancy to prevent blood vacuity:
Combine fresh chicken with carrots, parsley, a small amount of fresh ginger, possibly egg yolk, soybean sprouts, and water. Simmer for about three hours or more. Eat three to four times a week.

- *Stomach qi and spleen qi vacuity:*
  General lack of strength; loss of strength follow-

ing long, draining illness; infirmity in old age, decreased appetite, indigestion, diarrhea, edema

- *Stomach cold or spleen yang vacuity:*
  Sensation of cold in body, especially in stomach region, cold extremities, lack of appetite
- *General vacuity of kidney network:*
  Weakness and pain in knees and hip, premature ejaculation, tinnitus, frequent urination

Chicken boiled in rice wine with ginger and pepper

Contraindications

- *Restraint with general heat symptoms, especially heat in blood:*
  Skin disorders with reddened, raised, itching efflorescence
- *Restraint during beginning colds:*
  Pulls pathogenic factors into deeper layers

Chicken Liver

Preferably from organically raised animals.

Thermal nature	Warm
Flavor	Sweet
Organ network	Kidney, liver
Direction	Upbearing
Phase	Earth
Effect	Supplements liver, kidneys, *qi*, and blood
Preparation methods	Steamed, fried, or grilled
Contains	Protein, rich in vitamins and minerals

Indications

- *Kidney yang vacuity:*
  Weakness, back pains, impotence, nocturnal urination, cold extremities
- *Kidney blood vacuity:*
  Night blindness, insomnia, blurred vision, dizziness, numbness in extremities, muscle weakness

Steamed or fried chicken liver combined with lamb's lettuce (Mache lettuce), spinach, arugula, parsley, and mangold chard

Duck

Thermal nature	Neutral to cool
Flavor	Sweet and salty
Organ network	Lung, kidneys, stomach, spleen
Direction	Upbearing
Phase	Earth
Effect	Nourishes yin, supplements blood, strengthens stomach, moistens lung, clears heat, diuretic, reduces swelling.
Preparation methods	Fried, boiled, steamed, or as soup
Contains	Protein, fat, iron, vitamin B_1 and B_2

Indications

- *General yin vacuity with heat symptoms, especially lung yin vacuity:*
  Subfebrile temperatures, thirst, agitation, night sweat, dry mouth and throat, persisting cough with little phlegm

Braised or boiled duck

- *Spleen vacuity with fluid accumulation and edema:*

Braised duck stuffed with about half a cup of fresh ginger and one to three cloves of garlic to taste

- *Blood vacuity and general yin vacuity with yang hyperactivity:*
  Following high blood loss, for example after

childbirth; blurred vision, heart palpitations, sleep disturbances, headaches, rotatory vertigo

Duck and chicken soup with parsley and 50 g (about 2 oz) of brown seaweed (dry weight)

Contraindications
- Qi stagnation
- Spleen vacuit

Lamb, Mutton, Sheep

Thermal nature	Warm to hot
Flavor	Sweet
Organ network	Spleen, kidney
Direction	Upbearing/floating
Phase	Earth
Effect	Warms center burner and kidney network, supplements *qi* and blood, supports jing
Preparation methods	Steamed, fried/roasted, grilled, boiled
Contains	Protein, fat, calcium, phosphorus

Indications
- Lamb is especially recommended during the cold months as a warming food, served well spiced.
- *Very good for kidney yang vacuity:*
  Feeling of coldness in body, cold extremities, aversion to cold, weakness or pain in legs, back, or knees, increase of symptoms with cold, weak libido, impotence, frequent nocturnal urination with clear urine

Lamb fried/roasted, grilled or well-cooked in liquid with ginger, Chinese leek (garlic chives), walnuts, garlic, and carrots, preferably seasoned with rosemary, thyme, and oregano

- *Blood vacuity with cold symptoms after childbirth:*
  Abdominal pains, reduced milk flow, cold lower extremities

Lamb with fresh ginger

- *Stomach and spleen yang vacuity:*
  Lack of appetite, exhaustion, persistent chills, cold extremities, fatigue

Contraindications
- *Heat symptoms:*
  Agitation, insomnia, reddened itching skin disorders, excessive menstrual bleeding

Pork

Thermal nature	Neutral
Flavor	Sweet, salty
Organ network	Spleen, stomach, kidney
Direction	Downbearing
Phase	Earth, water
Effect	Enriches yin, moistens dryness, supplements blood
Preparation methods	Boiled, fried/roasted, grilled, or as soup
Contains	Protein, fat, calcium, phosphorus, iron

Indications
- *Qi and blood vacuity:*
  Emaciation, lack of strength, muscle weakness
- *Liver and kidney yin vacuity:*
  Dry eyes, night sweat, hypomenorrhea (scant menstruation), weakness and pain in hip, back, and bones
- *Dryness:*
  Thirst, dry cough, mouth and throat dryness, dry skin

Contraindications
- *Excessive consumption leads to obesity*
- *Excessive consumption promotes the formation of dampness and phlegm*

- *Avoid with heat phlegm disorders:*
  Bronchitis, sinusitis
- *Avoid with qi stagnation*

Rabbit/Hare

Thermal nature	Cool, neutral
Flavor	Sweet
Organ network	Liver, large intestine, stomach, spleen
Direction	Floating
Phase	Earth, ambiguous, depending on source
Effect	Supplements center burner, supplements *qi*, cools blood
Preparation methods	Boiled, fried/roasted, or steamed
Contains	Rich in protein, minerals, little fat

Indications

- *Stomach spleen qi vacuity:*
  Fatigue, lack of strength, lack of appetite
- *Heat in stomach and large intestine:*
  Constipation, nausea, vomiting, ravenous appetite
- *Stomach yin vacuity:*
  Constipation, lack of appetite, mouth dryness

Contraindications

- *Cold symptoms in stomach and spleen*

Venison (Deer)

Thermal nature	Warm, hot
Flavor	Acrid, sweet
Organ network	Kidney
Direction	Upbearing/floating
Phase	Earth; ambiguous, depending on source
Effect	Strengthens *qi*, blood, and yang, especially kidney yang, moves blood
Preparation methods	Fried/roasted, braised, or boiled
Contains	Protein, fat, minerals

Indications

- Venison is an excellent tonic for the kidney network to strengthen kidney *yang*; it is primarily suitable for the cold season diet.
- *General qi and blood vacuity:*
  Especially lack of strength, emaciation, fatigue
- *Kidney yang vacuity:*
  Aversion to cold, constant chills; weakness and pain in lower back, knees and legs with worsening of symptoms with cold; weak libido, impotence, frequent nocturnal urination

Braised venison in red wine with garlic or ginger, carrots, and walnuts

Contraindications

- *Exercise caution with heat symptoms based on a yin vacuity to avoid yang hyperactivity:*
  Agitation, insomnia, sexual hyperactivity, sudden sweating, migraines, or irregular and strong menorrhagia (excess/prolonged menstruation)

Fish/Sea Food

Fish (sweet water) often has a sweet/salty flavor and a neutral to warm thermal nature. It is easy to digest and strengthens *qi*, blood, and *yang*, especially the center burner (stomach, spleen/pancreas) and the kidneys.

Seafood (fish and shellfish from the ocean) is mostly salty and has a cool to cold thermal nature. It affects the liver and kidney network and nourishes *yin*.

- To treat **repletion** (strong person, loud powerful voice, choleric features, extroverted, red tongue, possibly thick fur): Squid/octopus.
- To treat **vacuity** (weak person, weak quiet voice, often tired and exhausted, pale, swollen tongue, weak pulse): Eel, sardines, mussels, oysters.
- To treat **heat** (red tongue, rapid pulse, red face, reddened eyes, nervousness): Squid/octopus.
- To treat **cold** (pale, swollen tongue, weak, slow pulse, shivering, aversion to cold, worsening of condition and pain with cold): Trout, salmon, prawns, crayfish.
- To treat **dampness** (swellings, edema, chronic phlegm disorders, frontal sinusitis, bronchitis): Carp, mackerel.
- To treat **dryness** (dry mouth, lips and skin, constipation): Oysters.

Anchovies

Thermal nature	Neutral
Flavor	Sweet, salty
Organ network	Stomach, spleen
Phase	Earth
Effect	Supplements *qi* and blood, warms stomach and spleen
Preparation methods	Deep-fried, fried, grilled, boiled
Contains	Protein, fat, vitamin B_1 and B_2

Indications

- *Qi and yang vacuity of stomach and spleen:* Lack of appetite, lack of strength, indigestion

Contraindications

- *Heat conditions:* Especially skin disorders

Carp

Thermal nature	Neutral
Flavor	Sweet
Organ network	Spleen, kidney
Direction	Downbearing
Phase	Earth
Effect	Supplements stomach and spleen, supplements *qi* and blood, dispels dampness, downbears *qi*, reduces swelling
Preparation methods	Steamed, boiled
Contains	Rich in protein and vitamin D

Indications

- *Spleen qi vacuity and spleen yang vacuity:*
  Swelling, edema
- *Qi and blood vacuity:*
  Insufficient milk flow, during recovery, lack of strength
- *Lung network vacuity:*
  Chronic cough, sensation of fullness in chest, shortness of breath

Contraindications

- Skin disorders

Crab

Thermal nature	Cold
Flavor	Salty
Organ network	Liver, stomach
Phase	Water
Effect	Clears heat, moves blood, strengthens muscles, sinews, and bones

Indications

- *Blood stasis:*
  Pain after injuries to muscles, sinews, and bones (swelling, tears, fractures)
- *Abdominal pain following childbirth, to increase blood circulation*

Soak and boil crab in rice wine and eat throughout the day

Contraindications

- During pregnancy
- Skin disorders

Eel

Thermal nature	Neutral, warm
Flavor	Sweet
Organ network	Spleen, liver, kidneys
Direction	Upbearing
Phase	Water
Effect	Supplements *qi* and yang, regulates wind and dampness
Preparation methods	Fried, boiled, or in soup
Contains	Protein, high fat content, calcium, phosphorus

Indications

- *Qi and yang vacuity:*
  Weakness, exhaustion, shortness of breath
- *Wind and dampness disorders:*
  Pain and swelling in extremities, weakness in legs and hips (rheumatic complaints caused by wind-dampness)

Cook eel in rice wine with salt, vinegar, and a little fresh ginger

Contraindications

- *Phlegm disorders*
- *Diarrhea caused by spleen and stomach vacuity*

Herring

Thermal nature	Neutral
Flavor	Sweet
Organ network	Spleen, lung
Direction	Downbearing
Phase	Earth
Effect	Supplements *qi* of stomach, spleen, and lung
Preparation methods	Deep-fried, fried, grilled, boiled
Contains	Protein, fat, minerals

Indications

- *Qi vacuity of stomach and spleen:*
  Lack of appetite, weakness, chronic digestive problems
- *Lung qi vacuity:*
  Rapid exhaustion, perspiring easily, shortness of breath

Contraindications

- Skin disorders

Mackerel

Thermal nature	Neutral
Flavor	Sweet
Organ network	Stomach, liver
Direction	Floating
Phase	Earth
Effect	Supplements *qi* and blood, removes dampness

Indications

Swelling, edema, rheumatism (damp impediment or *shi bi*)

Mussels

Thermal nature	Warm, neutral
Flavor	Salty
Organ network	Liver, kidney
Direction	Downbearing
Phase	Water
Effect	Enriches yin and yang of liver and kidneys, nourishes jing and blood

Indications

- *Kidney yang vacuity:*
  Impotence, back pain, weak back

Mussels cooked in wine or rice wine with onions, leeks, carrots, garlic, and pepper

- *Yin vacuity:*
  Nocturnal sweating and dizziness

Oysters

Thermal nature	Neutral
Flavor	Sweet, salty
Organ network	Kidney, liver
Direction	Downbearing
Phase	Earth, water
Effect	Supplements *qi* and blood, nourishes blood, enriches yin and yang of kidneys, moistens dryness, cools blood.
Preparation methods	Raw, deep fried, simmered in liquid
Contains	Rich in minerals

Indications

- *Yin vacuity:*
  Sleep disturbance, nervousness, fluid vacuity, blood vacuity, excessive perspiration, night sweats, excessive alcohol consumption
- *Kidney network vacuity:*
  Exhaustion, premature ejaculation, spermatorrhea (involuntary discharge of semen)

Contraindications

- Skin disorders

Prawns/Crayfish/Lobster

Thermal nature	Warm
Flavor	Sweet
Organ network	Kidney, liver
Direction	Floating
Phase	Earth
Effect	Enriches yang, especially kidney yang; supplements *qi* and blood, dispels cold, disperses blood stasis, eliminates wind and phlegm
Preparation methods	Deep-fried, fried, grilled, boiled
Contains	Protein, minerals

Indications

- *Kidney yang vacuity:*
  Impotence, premature ejaculation, weak libido, lack of strength, pain in lumbar region.

Prawns fried in alcohol with garlic, ginger, and Chinese leeks (garlic chives)

- *Qi and blood vacuity:*
  After childbirth, stimulates milk flow and milk production

Contraindications

- *Blood heat disorders:*
  Can produce efflorescence with skin disorders

Sardines

Thermal nature	Neutral, warm
Flavor	Sweet, salty
Organ network	Stomach, spleen, kidneys
Direction	Upbearing
Phase	Earth, water
Effect	Supplements *qi*, *yang*, and blood; warms stomach and spleen, supplements kidneys
Preparation methods	Deep-fried, fried, grilled, boiled
Contains	Protein, fat, minerals

Indications

- *Stomach and spleen vacuity:*
  Lack of appetite, lack of strength, indigestion, edema
- *Kidney network vacuity:*
  Impotence, decreased libido, back pain and weakness, sinew and bone weakness

Grilled sardines with garlic

Contraindications

- Heat conditions
- Skin disorders

Squid, Octopus

Thermal nature	Cold
Flavor	Sweet, salty
Organ network	Kidney, bladder, liver
Direction	Downbearing
Phase	Water
Effect	Nourishes yin, strengthens blood and *qi*, clears heat
Preparation methods	Deep-fried, fried, grilled, boiled
Contains	Protein, fat, minerals

Indications

- *Yang vacuity and heat conditions rooted in liver yin vacuity or kidney yin vacuity:*
  Dizziness, tinnitus, sudden profuse menorrhagia (menstrual bleeding), strong menstrual pain with light-red blood
- *Blood heat:*
  Itching skin disorders
- *Stomach heat caused by liver repletion:*
  Heartburn, gastritis, gastric and duodenal ulcers

Contraindications

- *With heat symptoms avoid:*
  Deep-fried, fried, or grilled

Trout

Thermal nature	Warm, hot
Flavor	Sweet
Organ network	Stomach, spleen
Direction	Upbearing/floating
Phase	Wood
Effect	Enriches yang, regulates *qi*, dispels cold, warms stomach and spleen
Preparation methods	Boiled, grilled, fried
Contains	Protein, minerals

Indications

- *Stomach and spleen vacuity:*
  Lack of appetite, general weakness, bloating, diarrhea
- *Qi and yang vacuity:*
  Weakness, exhaustion, cold extremities, shortness of breath

Grilled trout with garlic and almonds

Contraindications

- Wind–heat disorders
- Rashes

Tuna

Due to its high degree of metal toxicity (higher than most other fish), tuna is not recommended during nutritional therapy, and possibly also afterward.

Dairy Products, Eggs, Oils, and Fats

Milk and dairy products are considerably less prevalent in Chinese nutrition than in the Western world. They are sweet in flavor and neutral to cold in thermal nature; they moisten dryness and enrich *yin*. Excessive consumption, often found in our "modern diet," can quickly lead to phlegm disorders (recurrent colds with phlegm production, frontal sinusitis, bronchitis, chronic headaches with heaviness and dull pressure).

The center burner especially suffers when "overfed" with dairy products, and produces dampness and eventually phlegm disorders in the body. Children are especially at risk from excess dairy products, often in combination with other cold foods (citrus fruits and juices) and overly fatty, phlegm-forming foods (sugary sodas, junk food). In children under age eight, the center burner is not yet fully developed, which makes it difficult for them to compensate for excess cold, cool, dampness, and phlegm-producing foods.

For cheeses, the harder a cheese, the less dampness, it will generate (if eaten in moderation!) and the warmer it is in temperature. Cottage cheese, for example, is cool, while Parmesan is neutral to warm in thermal nature.

Fats and oils are mostly of neutral thermal nature when raw, but change to warm/hot when heated (deep-frying). They moisten dryness (constipation) and nourish *yin*. Excessive consumption causes dampness and phlegm, or hot phlegm from deep-frying oils.

Caution: Avoid dairy products and oils in case of spleen *qi* and spleen *yang* vacuity!

- To treat **repletion** (robust person, loud, powerful voice, sensation of heat, hyperactivity, choleric features, extroverted, tongue with thick fur, replete pulse): Yogurt in moderation.
- To treat **vacuity** (weak person; weak, quiet voice; shivering, frequent fatigue and exhaustion, introverted, swollen tongue, weak pulse) (to treat *yin* vacuity): Butter, cream, cheese, milk, eggs.
- To treat **heat** (red face, craving for cold drinks; worsening of symptoms from cold; pale, swollen tongue; weak, slow pulse): Avoid dairy products!
- To treat **dampness** (general sensation of heaviness, pathological swelling, edema; chronic phlegm disorders, e.g., frontal sinusitis, bronchitis, cysts, tumors): Avoid dairy products!
- To treat **dryness** (dry mouth, lips, and chapped skin; dry mucous membranes): Butter, cream, oils, cheese, milk.

Pasteurized dairy products are warmer in thermal nature than raw milk, cream, or cheese made from raw milk. Some nutritional components in milk are lost when milk is heated above body temperature.

Butter and Cream

Butter produces less dampness than cream.

Thermal nature	Warm, neutral
Flavor	Sweet
Organ network	Spleen, liver, lung, kidney, large intestine
Direction	Upbearing
Phase	Earth
Effect	Supplements *qi*, yin, and blood; moistens dryness, disperses blood stasis
Preparation methods	Raw or in cooking
Contains	Rich in protein, fat, carbohydrates, minerals

Indications

- *Qi vacuity:*
  Fatigue, exhaustion, mental exhaustion
- *Yin vacuity:*
  Dry mouth and throat, dry cough, dry skin, constipation, nervousness

Contraindications

- *Avoid with blood heat disorders:*
  Itching skin disorders
- *Excess can weaken spleen and cause dampness and phlegm disorders:*
  More pronounced with cream

Cow's Milk

Thermal nature	Neutral, cool
Flavor	Sweet
Organ network	Lung, stomach, heart
Direction	Upbearing
Phase	Earth
Effect	Supplements *qi*, *yin*, and blood; supplements lung, stomach, and heart; creates body fluids, moistens intestine and skin, detoxifies
Preparation methods	Raw, boiled, in porridge
Contains	Rich in protein, minerals and vitamins, calcium, phosphorus, iron, vitamins A, B_1, B_2, B6, and C.

Indications

- *General qi and blood vacuity:*
  Weakness, mental exhaustion, dizziness, overexertion, consumption (especially in old age)

Milk porridge.
Simmer 100 g (half a cup) of cooked short-grain (glutinous) rice in about 0.5 L (two cups) of milk. Add cinnamon and raisins.

- *Stomach yin vacuity:*
  Dry mouth and throat, lack of appetite, constipation

Fresh milk boiled with a little ginger juice

Contraindications

- *Excessive consumption of milk and milk products can easily weaken the stomach and spleen network and often leads to dampness and phlegm disorders, especially in children:*
  Dull, heavy head, lack of concentration, chronic fatigue, loose stool, diarrhea, recurrent infections: colds, bronchitis, sinusitis, ear infections

Cow's Milk Cheese

Thermal nature	Neutral, cool (blue cheese: warm)
Flavor	Sweet, sour
Organ network	Stomach, spleen, lung, liver
Direction	Upbearing and downbearing
Phase	Wood, earth
Effect	Supplements and moves *qi*, nourishes yin, moistens, laxative
Preparation methods	Raw or melted
Contains	Rich in fat and protein, minerals

Indications

- *Yin vacuity, especially lung yin vacuity:*
  Dry cough, sore throat, hoarseness, dry skin, night sweats
- *Dryness in large intestine:*
  Constipation

Contraindications

- *Cheese, especially blue cheese, can cause dampness and phlegm disorders when eaten in excess*

Chicken Eggs

Thermal nature	Raw: neutral, cool Cooked: warm
Flavor	Sweet
Organ network	Egg white: lung Egg yolk: heart, kidney
Direction	Upbearing
Phase	Earth
Effect	Supplements *qi* and blood, nourishes yin, moistens, calms the fetus Egg white: moistens lung, clears heat Egg yolk: enriches yin and blood, moistens
Preparation methods	Raw, boiled, fried, scrambled
Contains	Rich in protein, fat, especially lecithin, cholesterol and triglycerides, as well as vitamin A and D, iron, phosphorus

Indications

- *Qi vacuity:*
  (Egg yolk!) exhaustion, weakness, fatigue, during recovery, malnutrition
- *Yin and blood vacuity:*
  Nervousness, sleep disorders, heart palpitations, dizziness, night blindness
- *Lung yin vacuity:*
  Sore throat, hoarseness, dry cough, loss of voice
- *Stomach yin vacuity:*
  Lack of appetite
- *Heat symptoms:*
  (Egg white!) reddened eyes, strong movement of fetus, thirst after delivery

Contraindications

Excess causes

- *Wind disorders:*
  Skin rashes
- *Qi stagnation*
- *Moist–heat*

Goat's and Sheep's Milk

Thermal nature	Warm
Flavor	Sweet
Organ network	Lung, stomach, in part heart and kidneys
Direction	Upbearing
Phase	Earth
Effect	Warms and moistens stomach and spleen
Preparation methods	Raw or cooked
Contains	Rich in protein, fat, minerals, especially calcium and phosphorus

Indications

- *General qi vacuity:*
  Fatigue, weakness, indigestion, emaciation
- *Stomach yin vacuity:*
  Dry mouth and throat, lack of appetite, constipation

Goat's and Sheep's Milk Cheese

Thermal nature	Warm, neutral
Flavor	Sweet, sour, salty
Organ network	Stomach, spleen, lung, liver, heart, kidneys
Direction	Upbearing and downbearing
Phase	Wood, earth
Effect	Supplements and moves *qi*, warms stomach and spleen, nourishes yin
Preparation methods	Raw or melted
Contains	Rich in fat and protein, minerals

Indications

- *Stomach and spleen vacuity:*
  Indigestion
- *Dryness in large intestine:*
  Constipation

Contraindications

- *Excessive consumption can cause dampness and phlegm disorders*

Peanut Oil

Thermal nature	Neutral
Flavor	Sweet
Organ network	Large intestine, lung, stomach
Direction	Upbearing
Phase	Earth
Effect	Supplements center burner, moistens lung and large intestine, antiparasitic
Preparation methods	For frying and deep-frying
Contains	High-quality essential fatty acids, especially the heart-friendly linoleic acid, B-vitamins

Indications

- *Stomach spleen vacuity:*
  Lack of appetite
- *Dryness in lung or large intestine:*
  Dry cough with little sputum, constipation

Contraindications

- Excess leads to formation of phlegm

Sesame Oil

Thermal nature	Cool
Flavor	Sweet
Organ network	Large intestine, liver, kidney
Direction	Downbearing
Phase	Earth
Effect	Moistens intestines, laxative, detoxifies
Preparation methods	As a seasoning or for salads, sparingly for occasional frying
Contains	High in unsaturated fatty acids, lecithin, vitamin E

Indications

- *Dryness in intestines:*
  Constipation, digestive obstructions
- *Blood and qi vacuity of liver and kidney:*
  Weakness in muscles, sinews, and bones

Contraindications

Excess
- *Weakens the spleen/pancreas network*
- Can cause diarrhea

Soybean Oil

Thermal nature	Warm
Flavor	Acrid and sweet
Organ network	Large intestine
Direction	Upbearing
Phase	Earth, metal
Effect	Moistens intestines, disperses blood stasis, laxative, antiparasitic
Preparation methods	For frying and deep-frying
Contains	High amounts of unsaturated fatty acids, linolenic acid, oleic acid, rich in vitamin E; cold-pressed soy bean oil is similar to wheat germ oil in potency and quality

Indications

- Constipation

Yogurt

Thermal nature	Cool, cold
Flavor	Sweet, sour
Organ network	Liver, lungs, large intestine (ambiguous, depending on sources)
Direction	Downbearing
Phase	Earth, wood
Effect	Nourishes yin, clears heat, relaxes liver, moistens lung, quenches thirst
Preparation methods	Raw
Contains	Protein, fat, carbohydrates, minerals

Indications

- *Heat symptoms:*
  Restlessness, nervousness, sleep disturbances, thirst
- *Stomach heat:*
  Pain in epigastric region, gastritis, stomach ulcers, heartburn
- *Heat in liver, upbearing liver yang:*
  Restlessness, irritability, sudden temporal headaches, dizziness, red itching eyes
- *Dryness and heat in intestine:*
  Constipation
- *External use:*
  Skin eruption with itching, rough, dry skin from sunburn

Contraindications

- *Cold symptoms in center burner*
- Diarrhea
- *If eaten in excess, risk of dampness and phlegm formation*

Nuts and Seeds

Nuts and seeds are highly nutritious and mostly warm in thermal nature. They are ideal for building up *qi* and *yang* in the body. Nuts can quickly balance energy deficiencies (e.g., "energy balls" made with walnuts, honey, and coconut).

- To treat **repletion** (robust person; loud, powerful voice; sensation of heat, hyperactivity, choleric features, extroverted, tongue with thick fur, replete pulse): White sesame.
- To treat **vacuity:** (weak person; weak, quiet voice; shivering, frequently tired and exhausted; introverted, swollen tongue, weak pulse): Walnuts, peanuts, pine nuts, chestnuts.
- To treat **heat** (red face, thirst for cold drinks, worsening of symptoms and pain from heat, red tongue, rapid pulse): Avoid nuts and seeds, instead choose fresh sprouts (mung beans).
- To treat **cold** (shivering, aversion to cold, worsening of condition and pain from cold; pale, swollen tongue; weak, slow pulse): Walnuts, chestnuts.
- To treat **dryness** (dry mouth, lips and chapped skin, dry mucous membranes): Sunflower seeds.

Almonds

Thermal nature	Neutral
Flavor	Sweet
Organ network	Lung, large intestine, spleen
Direction	Upbearing
Phase	Earth
Effect	Moistens lung, relieves cough, transforms phlegm, downbears *qi*, moistens large intestine
Preparation methods	Raw, roasted, ground, and as decoction
Contains	Rich in fats, protein, calcium, iron, magnesium, phosphorus, potassium, relatively high amount of vitamin A; also C, B-complex, enzymes with hormone character

Indications

- *Dryness and lung vacuity:*
  Cough with breathing problems, wheezing, dry mouth and throat

Mix ground almonds, ground walnuts, and honey dissolved in warm water

- *Dryness in large intestine:*
  Constipation
- *Spleen vacuity:*
  Lack of appetite, lack of strength

Contraindications

- *Dampness and phlegm disorders*

Black Sesame

Thermal nature	Neutral to cool; roasted sesame is thermally much warmer than raw sesame
Flavor	Sweet
Organ network	Liver, kidney
Direction	Downbearing
Phase	Earth
Effect	Supplements liver and kidney, moistens dryness
Preparation methods	Raw, roasted, ground, cooked with liquid as porridge, as a seasoning, or made into butter
Contains	Rich in essential fatty acids, carbohydrates, protein, phosphorus, vitamin E, calcium, iron, phosphorus, selenium, silicic acid, lecithin

Indications

- *Liver and kidney vacuity:*
  General lack of strength, weakness in knees and back, muscle pain, weakness in extremities, tinnitus, rotary vertigo, impotence
- *Blood vacuity and exhaustion of fluids:*
  Postpartum lactation problems; dizziness, forgetfulness
- *Wind impediments (feng bi):*
  Rheumatic disorders (arthritis), dry cough, dryness in large intestine: constipation

Roasted sesame to strengthen blood and kidneys:
Roast black sesame in a dry pan until fragrant; eat one to two teaspoons daily

Black sesame porridge:
Mix 50 g (half a cup) of black sesame seeds and 100 g (half a cup) of short-grain (glutinous) rice with water and simmer for about 20–30 minutes

- *Balances liver and kidneys, strengthens muscles, sinews, and bones, for weakness in arms, legs, and back*

Contraindications

- Diarrhea
- *Use cautiously with heat symptoms*

Chestnut

Thermal nature	Warm
Flavor	Sweet
Organ network	Stomach, spleen, kidney
Direction	Upbearing
Phase	Earth
Effect	Supplements kidneys, supplements *qi* and blood, disperses *qi* stagnation, dispels cold, strengthens sinews and muscles, balances stomach and spleen
Preparation methods	Raw, roasted, as porridge or decoction
Contains	Less fat and protein than other types of nuts, also calcium, phosphorus, potassium, sulfur, magnesium, iron, carotene, vitamin B_1, B_2, C, and E

Indications

- *Kidney vacuity:*
  Weakness and pain in hip, knees, and lower back

Roasted chestnuts or as a porridge with walnuts

- *Yang vacuity of spleen and kidney:*
  Diarrhea, cold extremities, lack of strength, impotence, back pain

Roasted chestnuts

- *External application:*
  For injuries, swelling due to blocked blood flow

Contraindications

- Excessive consumption leads to bloating and abdominal distention

Hazelnut

Thermal nature	Neutral
Flavor	Sweet
Organ network	Spleen, stomach
Direction	Upbearing
Phase	Earth
Effect	Harmonizes center burner, regulates *qi*
Preparation methods	Raw, roasted, ground, or as nut butter
Contains	High amount of fat, thus high percentage of unsaturated fatty acids, protein, carbohydrates, calcium, iron, phosphorus, magnesium, sulfur, rich in B-vitamins, vitamin C, tannins (stimulate skin and intestinal function), high lecithin content

Indications

- Spleen/pancreas organ network vacuity: Lack of appetite, fatigue

Peanut

Thermal nature	Neutral *Raw:* cool *Roasted or boiled:* warm
Flavor	Sweet
Organ network	Spleen, lung
Direction	Upbearing
Phase	Earth
Effect	Supplements center burner, harmonizes stomach, moistens lung, relieves cough, promotes milk production, moistens large intestine
Preparation methods	Raw, roasted, boiled or ground
Contains	Extremely high protein and fat content, rich in B-vitamins. Note: large amounts of linoleic acid, vitamin E, potassium, magnesium, calcium, zinc, phosphorus, manganese, most essential amino acids—plenty of tryptophane (important for sleeping!)

Indications

- *Spleen vacuity:*
  Lack of appetite, lack of strength

Decoction of 60 g (about one quarter cup) each of peanuts, adzuki beans, and jujube beans boiled in water, taken throughout the day.

- *Dryness and lung vacuity:*
  Dry cough with little sputum, dry throat, persistent cough

Mixture of peanut butter and almond butter, mixed with honey

- *Dryness in large intestine:*
  Constipation
- *Qi and blood vacuity:*
  After childbirth with reduced milk flow

Contraindications
- Excess produces dampness, phlegm, and diarrhea

Pine Nuts

Thermal nature	Neutral, tendency to warm
Flavor	Sweet
Organ network	Lung, liver, large intestine
Direction	Upbearing
Phase	Earth
Effect	Moistens lung and large intestine, creates body fluids, expels wind and cold
Preparation methods	Raw, roasted, as a paste or pill
Contains	Rich in essential fatty acids, calcium, phosphorus, iron, highest in vitamin B_1 of all nuts

Indications
- *Dryness and lung vacuity:*
  Dry throat, cough with little or no phlegm, recurrent cough

Porridge of ground pine nuts (30 g or about two tablespoons) and ground walnuts (60 g or about half a cup) mixed with honey (20 g or one teaspoon)

- *Dryness in large intestine:*
  Constipation
- *Wind impediment (feng bi) or internal liver wind:*
  Rheumatism (arthritis), dizziness, drowsiness

Contraindications
- *Excess can cause dampness and phlegm production*

Sunflower Seeds

Thermal nature	Neutral
Flavor	Sweet
Organ network	Lung, large intestine
Direction	Upbearing
Phase	Earth
Effect	Supplements spleen, enriches yin, moistens large intestine
Preparation methods	Raw, roasted, or as oil
Contains	Rich in fats and essential fatty acids, especially linoleic acid and lecithin, protein, carbohydrates, vitamin B_1, B_2, and D as well as calcium, iron

Indications
- *Spleen/pancreas network vacuity*:
  Lack of drive, lack of strength, diarrhea
- Hyperlipidemia (high cholesterol), high blood pressure, arteriosclerosis (Western and Chinese medicine)

Contraindications
- *Caution with heat symptoms*

Alcoholic Beverages, Coffee, and Tea

Alcoholic Beverages

Thermal nature	Dependent on alcohol content: the more high-proof, the warmer or hotter. *Brandy:* hot *Wine:* warm *Beer:* cool, especially wheat beer (during summer heat)
Flavor	Acrid, sweet, and bitter
Organ network	Heart, liver, lung, stomach
Direction	Upbearing
Phase	Metal
Effect	Moves *qi*, moves blood, dispels cold, disperses liver *qi* stagnation
Preparation methods	Consumed in small amounts, for preserving and seasoning foods
Contains	Ethanol, fatty acid, acids, possibly sugar

Indications

- *Short-term qi vacuity:*
  Fatigue, exhaustion (decoction of alcohol and *radix ginseng*)
- *Blood stasis and cold:*
  Cold extremities, shivering, pain in abdomen
- *Blood vacuity:*
  Pale complexion, insomnia, forgetfulness, fatigue
- (Red wine in moderation also strengthens kidney energy, pain and tension in lower back region)
- *Liver qi stagnation:*
  Mental and physical tension, depression, melancholy, dysmenorrhea (lack of menstruation)
- *Invasion of wind–cold:*
  Aversion to cold, shivering, pain in extremities, pain in chest and back

Alcohol balances *qi*, strengthens lung, spleen, and heart networks.
In combination with the appropriate herbs, alcohol can have an accelerating and strengthening effect. The colder seasons are preferable for treatments using alcohol.

Basic recipe for medicinal wines/liqueurs:

Immerse individual herbs or herb combinations in clear, high-proof alcohol (e.g., rice wine, gin, vodka) for at least two weeks and up to several months.

Example
Ginseng liqueur (*radix ginseng* [Latin]/ *Ren Chen* [Chinese]).
Immerse root in clear, high-proof alcohol for at least six weeks; second brew possible.

Contraindications

- *Liver yin vacuity*
- *Heat symptoms*
- *Damp–heat*
- *Regular excessive alcohol consumption damages qi, damages the spirit (shen), and destroys yin.*

Coffee

Thermal nature	Warm to hot
Flavor	Bitter and sweet
Direction	Upbearing
Phase	Fire
Effect	Warms and strengthens heart, stimulant, stimulates mental capacities, diuretic, detoxifies after excessive alcohol consumption, dries out body fluids
Preparation methods	Pour boiling water over ground coffee beans, possibly add milk and sugar
Contains	Sucrose, polysaccharide, fat, protein, caffeine potassium

Indications

- *General qi and yang vacuity:*
  Fatigue, exhaustion, sensation of cold inside body, headaches, dizziness, especially of the heart
- *After alcohol abuse*
- *Spleen yang vacuity:*
  Fatigue, indigestion, cold extremities

Contraindications

- *Coffee dries out body fluids, can lead to blood vacuity and, when consumed in excess, can permanently damage the kidney network.*

Consumed in small amounts (about one to two cups), coffee is therapeutic.
Negative effects appear when overdosed or with daily excessive consumption (four or more cups).

Tip: To alleviate the diuretic, dehydrating effect of coffee, drink a glass of water with each cup ("coffee culture" in Austria and Italy).

Tea

The effect of tea depends on the type of tea, processing, and preparation. A basic distinction can be made between fermented black tea and unfermented green or white tea. Green tea is preferred for medicinal purposes in China.

Thermal nature	Green and white tea: cool to cold; Black tea: cool to slightly warming
Flavor	Bitter and sweat
Organ network	Stomach, lung, heart, kidneys
Phase	Wood, earth, fire (not clear)
Effect	Clears heat, especially in head region; quenches thirst, diuretic, downbears *qi*, disperses digestive obstruction, refreshes the mind, transforms phlegm and dampness, detoxifies, harmonizes stomach (black tea)
Preparation methods	Brewed, powdered, and as decoction
Contains	Caffeine, tannins, essential oils, vitamin C and carotene, vitamin B_1 and B_2, minerals

Indications

- *Wind-cold disorders:*
  Aching, itchy eyes; blurred vision, headaches, heat sensation and dizziness in head
- *Summer heat with strong thirst*
- *Heat symptoms:*
  Thirst, nervousness, agitation, after excessive alcohol consumption
- *Damp-heat disorders:*
  Diarrhea or dysentery
- *Damp-heat:*
  Fatigue, exhaustion, heavy extremities
- *Heat symptoms:*
  Agitation, nervousness, after excessive alcohol consumption

- *Internal wind–heat:*
  Sensation of heat in head, dizziness, blurred vision, headaches and aching eyes

Contraindications

- *Cold and vacuity of stomach and spleen*
- *Sleep disturbances*
- *Excess dries out body fluids, especially blood (xue). Exercise caution with blood vacuity!*

5 Clinical Examples

Analogy of Western Diagnoses with Syndromes in Traditional Chinese Medicine (TCM)

Any form of treatment for the disorders above, including the use of nutritional therapy, needs to be preceded by a clear diagnosis by a trained TCM practitioner.
Treatment should never take place without a prior consultation with the treating physician.
The analogies between Western diagnoses and syndromes in TCM are not limited to the disorders discussed in this book. These are intended as a starting point for connecting Eastern and Western medical systems.

Respiratory Tract Disorders

Main Symptom: Colds

Acute cases of flu	*Wind–cold fettering the lung (feng han shu fei)*
Acute bronchitis	*Wind–heat invading the lung (feng re fan fei)*
Bronchitis, sinusitis, with yellow secretion	*Phlegm–heat obstructing the lung (tan re zu fei)*

According to TCM:
Cough (ke sou) and phlegm–rheum (tan yin) develop through the assault of external pathogenic factors, mostly cold, which block the flow of qi. These primarily occur due to lung, spleen, and kidney vacuity.

Nutritional therapy, along with acupuncture and herbal therapy, can produce very good results during the onset, as well as the subsequent course of the disorder.

■ Acute Case of Flu

Wind–Cold Fettering the Lung (Feng Han Shu Fei)
Wind–Cold Cough (Feng Han Ke Sou)

Symptoms

Stuffy or runny nose, with clear, watery phlegm, sneezing, cough, aversion to cold, aching limbs, headache, sore throat.

Tongue: Thin white fur
Pulse: Superficial, weak

Causes

External invasion of wind–cold into the lung due to weak defense *qi*. Lung function and flow of *qi* are impaired by cold.

Therapy

Clear body surface
激 • LU-7 • BL-12 • LI-4

Expel wind and cold
激 • TB-5 • GB-20 • SI-14

Avoid:
Raw, cold, and cool foods, and dairy products (they encourage phlegm disorders).

Recommended:

Thermal nature	Hot and warm
Organ network	Lung, spleen/pancreas
Direction	Floating
Preparation methods	Boiled, fried
Flavor	Acrid
Vegetables	Green onions, coriander
Beverages	Spiced tea, mulled wine, grog (beverage with rum, hot water, and sugar), whis-key
Spices	Aniseed, chili, ginger, garlic, pepper, rosemary, thyme (loosens phlegm, disinfects), cinnamon

Ginger tea:
Place thumb-sized pieces of ginger in 0.5 L (two cups) of water, simmer for about 20 minutes; drink while warm; add licorice for sore throat

Mulled wine

Spiced tea
(Yogi tea with pepper, ginger, cardamom, and cinnamon)

At the first onset of sneezing, shivering, and cold symptoms, expel cold and wind with hot and spicy foods for one day.

Decoction of spring onions and ginger

Chili con carne

As soon as symptoms shift from wind–cold to wind–heat (possibly overnight), with the predominant symptom of fever with sweating, immediately change nutritional therapy and choose cool and cold foods.

Acute Bronchitis

Wind–Heat Invading the Lung (Feng Re Fan Fei)

Symptoms

Burning sore throat, frequent cough, yellow secretion, fever, aversion to cold, stuffy nose, aching body and aching limbs, headaches.

Tongue: Thin yellow fur
Pulse: Superficial, fast

Causes

Wind–heat attacks on the lung, summer flu, weakened defense *qi* or next stage of a wind–cold attack on the lung (transformation from cold to heat can occur within a few hours).

Therapy

Clear surface
Dispel wind–heat
激
- LU-5 • LI-4 • LI-11 • GB-20
- BL-13 • LU-11 (for sore throat)
- ST-40 (for secretion)

Avoid:
Warm and hot foods, dairy products (encourage congestion).

Recommended:

Thermal nature	Cool, possibly a little cold
Phase	Metal, earth
Flavor	Acrid, bitter, possibly a little sweet
Preparation methods	Raw, boiled, steamed
Fruit	Pears, watermelons
Vegetables	Chinese (napa) cabbage, mung beans (sprouts even cooler), radish, black soybeans, dandelion
Beverages	Pear juice (for dryness, sore throat, and phlegm), green tea, peppermint tea
Grains	Wheat
Spices	Chinese chrysanthemum blossoms, mulberry leaves, salt /salt water
Soy products	Tofu

Relief during initial stage:
Concentrated peppermint tea, Chinese chrysanthemum blossom tea

Dry cough:
Pear juice

Sore throat:
Figs, fresh lemon juice

Cough relief and loosening of phlegm:
Roasted almonds with salt

Cough and loss of voice:
Fresh radish juice and ginger

■ Bronchitis, Sinusitis with Yellow Secretion

Phlegm–Heat Obstructing the Lung (Tan Re Zu Fei)

Symptoms

Cough with copious yellow, possibly green, sputum; bloating and feeling of pressure in chest, exhaustion, lack of appetite, soft stools.
Tongue: Red, with thick, sticky, yellow fur
Pulse: Fast, slippery

Causes

Long-term damage or constitutional vacuity of lung *qi*, combined with a spleen *qi* vacuity, promotes the formation of dampness and phlegm; inappropriate diet, excess of fatty, hot dishes.

Therapy

Loosen phlegm
Clear heat
激 • LU-7 • LU-5 • LI-4 • LI-11 • BL-13
• ST-40 (transforms phlegm)

Avoid:

Dairy products (promote congestion), bananas, alcoholic beverages, reduce consumption of meat.

Recommended:

Thermal nature	Neutral and cool, later neutral and warm to supplement the spleen
Organ network	Lung, spleen
Flavor	Slightly acrid, slightly sweet, salty (transforms phlegm)
Preparation methods	Raw, boiled, steamed
Mucolytic (decongesting) and transforming:	
Fruit	Pears, lemons
Beverages	Green tea
Grains	Soybeans
Vegetables	Bamboo sprouts, radish, red marine algae (dulse)
Cooling effect on lung:	
Vegetables	Bamboo sprouts, watercress, radish, celery root (celeriac), asparagus
Beverages	Peppermint tea, green and black tea
Supplement spleen and remove dampness:	
Grains	Millet, rice
Cough with phlegm:	
Vegetables	Button or crimini/portobella mushrooms
Nuts and seeds	Pine nuts, salt-roasted almonds

Tip: **Recurrent bronchial and sinus "phlegm conditions" respond very well to reducing the consumption of dairy products and meat.**

Bronchitis/Chronic Bronchitis

Chronic lung function impairment; recurrent bronchitis/chronic bronchitis	*Lung qi vacuity*
Chronic bronchitis with phlegm production (and phlegm retention in lung)	*Lung qi or spleen qi vacuity*
Chronic bronchitis with constitutional lung function impairment	*Lung yin and kidney yin vacuity*

According to TCM:
Cough "ke sou" and phlegm "tan yin" are caused by chronic vacuity of lung, spleen, and kidney. Treatment should primarily consist of acupuncture and herbal therapy, accompanied by dietary measures. Over a longer period (weeks to months), nutritional therapy can noticeably strengthen organ function and reduce formation of phlegm.

Chronic bronchitis is primarily a mixed syndrome of the above-mentioned primary syndromes. Treatment should target the primary syndrome. Treatment principles for nutritional therapy are supplementing the spleen for phlegm reduction and supplementing the lung and kidney to make up for chronic vacuity.

Chronic Lung Function Impairment; Recurrent Bronchitis/Chronic Bronchitis
Lung Qi Vacuity

Symptoms

Weak cough; thin, clear sputum; spontaneous perspiration, fatigue, susceptibility to infection.

Tongue: Pale
Pulse: Weak

Causes

Protracted and persistent cough weakens lung *qi*; constitutional weakness; general exhaustion (especially in old age).

Therapy

Supplement lung
激 • LU-9 • BL-13 • CV-6 • ST-36

Avoid:
Raw, cool, and cold foods, and bitter flavor.

Recommended:

Thermal nature	Neutral and warm
Organ network	Lung, spleen
Flavor	Slightly acrid, slightly sweet
Preparation methods	Boiled, steamed, fried
Meat	Duck
Fish	Carp
Fruit	Grapes
Vegetables	Cauliflower, carrots, onions
Grains	Oats, short-grain (glutinous) rice
Spices	Aniseed, ginger, garlic, rosemary, thyme
Nuts and seeds	Chestnuts, almonds, black sesame, sunflower seeds, walnuts
Other	Alcoholic beverages

Congee (see p. 117) with rice, onion, and ginger

Chronic Bronchitis with Phlegm Production (and Phlegm Retention in Lung)

Spleen Qi Vacuity and Lung Qi Vacuity

Symptoms

Cough with excessive white sputum, sensation of fullness in chest, fatigue, lack of appetite, soft stools.

Tongue: Whitish, slimy fur
Pulse: Slippery

Causes

Protracted or constitutional damage to lung *qi*, chronic spleen *qi* vacuity caused by inappropriate diet and overwork.

Therapy

Transform phlegm
Supplement spleen
Supplement lung
激 • LU-9 • BL-13 • ST-40 • CV-12
• PC-6 • SP-3 • BL-20

Avoid:
Raw, cold, and cool foods; dairy products, excess sweets, excess meat.

Recommended:
(see "Lung *Qi* Vacuity," p. 79)

Thermal nature	Neutral and warm
Organ network	Spleen, heart, lung
Flavor	Slightly sweet, slightly bitter, slightly acrid
Preparation methods	Boiled, fried, steamed
Transform phlegm:	
Fruit	Pears, cherries, apples
Vegetables	Leeks, radish
Grains	Millet
Spices	Ginger, garlic
Supplement spleen:	
Meat	Poultry, beef
Vegetables	Fennel, carrots
Grains	Oats, millet, rice
Spices	Aniseed, basil, ginger, coriander, thyme

Millet or rice dishes with acrid seasonings

■ Chronic Bronchitis, Constitutional Lung Disorder
Lung Yin Vacuity and Kidney Yin Vacuity

Symptoms

Dry cough, dry throat, chronic shortness of breath, weakness in knee and back, hot hands and feet, subfebrile temperatures in the afternoon.

Tongue: Red, dry, possibly no fur

Pulse: Thin

Causes

Protracted smoldering illness, chronic exhaustion, physiological process of aging.

Therapy

Supplement lung *yin* and kidney *yin*

激 • KI-3 • BL-23 • LU-7 • BL-13 • CV-4 • SI-4 • LU-9

Avoid:

Warm and hot foods, excess bitter and acrid flavor.

Recommended:

Thermal nature	Neutral and cool
Organ network	Lung, spleen, kidney
Flavor	Sweet, slightly salty
Preparation methods	Raw, steamed, boiled
Supplementing lung yin:	
Meat	Duck, pork
Fruit	Pears, tangerines, apricots, figs
Vegetables	Eggplant, button or crimini/portobella mushrooms, carrots, water chestnuts
Spices	Honey
Nuts and seeds	Peanuts, almonds, sunflower seeds, pine nuts
Dairy products	Butter, yogurt, farmer's cheese, cottage cheese, cow's milk
Soy products	Soy milk
Supplementing kidney yin:	
Meat	Duck, pork
Fish	Oysters, perch, octopus
Fruit	Cherries, grapes
Vegetables	Carrots
Grains	Wheat, corn
Nuts and seeds	Black sesame, walnuts
Other	Sheep's milk and goat's milk products

For dry cough:
Milk with honey, almond milk

Restorative soup with carrots and pork

Main Symptom: Cough

Acute weak cough	*Wind–cold fettering the lung (feng han shu fei)*
Acute violent cough	*Wind–heat invading the lung (feng re fan fei)*
Chronic cough with sputum	*Phlegm–damp cough* *(tan shi ke sou)*
Chronic dry cough	*Lung yin vacuity with dryness (fei yin xu, fei zao)*

According to TCM:
Counterflow lung qi; differential diagnosis based on frequency, severity, secretion and fever. Good results can be achieved with nutritional therapy, acupuncture, and herbs. Requires extended therapy over several weeks.

■ Acute Weak Cough

Wind–Cold Fettering the Lung (Feng Han Shu Fei)

Symptoms

Weak, quiet cough with thin white secretion, sore throat, fever without sweating, aversion to cold.

Therapy

Dispel wind and cold
Downbear *qi*
激 • LU-7 • BL-13 • TB-5
• LI-4 • GB-20 • ST-40

Avoid:
Cold and cool foods.

Recommended:

Beverages	Thyme tea with honey
Spices	Thyme, watercress, aniseed
Nuts and seeds	Roasted almonds with salt, walnuts with honey, almond butter

Aniseed tea

■ Acute Severe Cough

Wind–Heat Invading the Lung (Feng Re Fan Fei)

Symptoms

Frequent strong cough with yellow or greenish thin or viscous secretion, sore throat, fever, headaches.

Therapy

Expel wind and cold
激 • LU-5 • LU-11 • LI-4
• SI-14 • LI-11 • ST-40

Avoid:
Warm and hot foods.

Recommended:

Fruit	Pears, pear juice, grapefruit, lemons
Vegetables	Radish, bamboo sprouts
Beverages	Radish juice, green tea

Radish juice, pear juice, radish juice with ginger

Chronic Cough with Sputum

Phlegm–Damp Cough (Tan Shi Ke Sou)

Symptoms

Cough with excessive white sputum, exhaustion, bloating in thorax and epigastric region, loss of appetite.

Tongue: White, sticky fur

Pulse: Slippery

Causes

Chronic lung *qi* vacuity and spleen *qi* vacuity caused by external pathogenic factors and incorrect nutrition.

Therapy

Loosen phlegm

Supplement spleen *qi* and lung *qi*

激 • SP-3 + Moxa • LU-9 + Moxa • BL-13 + Moxa • BL-20 + Moxa • ST-40 • PC-6

Avoid:

Raw, cold, and cool foods, dairy products, meat, acrid and fatty foods, excess sweets.

Recommended:

Thermal nature	Neutral and warm
Organ network	Stomach, spleen, pancreas, lung
Flavor	Slightly sweet, bitter, acrid
Preparation methods	Raw, boiled
Fruit	Lemons, pears, apricots
Vegetables	Button or crimini/portobella mushrooms, fennel, radish, carrots, cauliflower, kohlrabi
Grains	Millet, rice, corn, oats
Spices	Ginger, aniseed, watercress, pepper
Nuts and seeds	Pine nuts, salted almonds, salted peanuts

Chronic Dry Cough

Lung Yin Vacuity with Dryness (Fei Yin Su, Fei Zao)

Symptoms

Persistent, dry, intense cough, little or no secretion, dry throat, thirst, fever in the afternoon, heat sensation in hands and feet.

Tongue: Red, dry, possibly thin, yellow fur

Pulse: Thin

Causes

Damage caused by external or internal heat, depletion of body fluids.

Therapy

Nourish *yin*

Dispel heat

Moisten dryness

激 • KI-6 • SP-5 • LU-6 • BL-13 • LU-9 • LU-7

Avoid:

Acrid and hot foods.

Recommended:

Thermal nature	Neutral, cool, and cold
Organ network	Stomach, spleen/pancreas, lung
Flavor	Sweet
Preparation methods	Boiled, steamed, baked (au gratin)
Meat	Duck, pork
Fruit	Pears
Beverages	Pear juice, aniseed tea
Spices	Honey, aniseed, watercress
Dairy products	Butter, cream
Nuts and seeds	Almond butter, pine nuts, sesame, walnuts with honey, peanuts
Soy products	Tofu, soymilk
Other	Chicken eggs

Peanut milk, peanut butter, and almond butter mixed with honey, paste of ground pine nuts, almonds, and walnuts.

Main Symptom: Sore Throat

Acute tonsillitis	*Wind–heat invading the lung (feng re fan fei)*
Acute laryngitis	*Wind–cold fettering the lung (feng han shu fei)*
Acute/chronic laryngitis	*Dryness–heat damaging the lung (zao re shang fei)*

According to TCM:
The most common cause of these disorders is attack of external pathogenic factors (wind–heat, wind–cold). Acute disorders are usually a repletion syndrome, whereas chronic illnesses generally appear as a vacuity syndrome. Acute disorders can be treated with good results by immediate application of acupuncture, nutritional therapy, and herbs.

Acute Tonsillitis

Wind–Heat Invading the Lung (Feng Re Fan Fei)

Symptoms
Painful reddened and swollen throat, burning pain, trouble swallowing, hoarseness, thirst, sometimes cough with thick yellow sputum; reddened swollen, possibly yellow–whitish tonsils.
Tongue: Yellow fur
Pulse: Superficial

Causes
Penetration of external wind and heat factors that deplete body fluids (summer heat, central heating, steel workers).

Therapy
Remove external pathogenic heat

Supplement lung
激
- LU-11 (microbleeding)
- LU-5 • LI-11
- LI-4 • GB-20 • LU-7 • ST-44

Avoid:
Foods with sour flavor, for example lemon, poultry (they draw pathogenic factors deeper into the body); foods with hot and warm thermal natures (too drying).

Recommended:

Thermal nature	Cool and cold
Organ network	Lung, spleen/pancreas
Flavor	Mildly acrid (to expel pathogenic factors, but avoid creating heat), sweet (moistens)
Preparation methods	Raw, boiled, steamed
For cooling:	
Fruit	Mulberries, watermelons, lemons, mangos
Vegetables	Dandelion, mung beans, radish, tomatoes
Beverages	Green tea
Grains	Wheat
Spices	Peppermint
To moisten dryness:	
Fruit	Pears
Beverages	Pear juice, melon juice, tomato juice

Mixture of tomato and watermelon juices. For dryness, drink pear juice with honey. Gargle with or drink fresh juice of one to two lemons.

■ Acute Laryngitis

Wind–Cold Fettering the Lung (Feng Han Shu Fei)

Symptoms

Scratchy throat, hoarseness, weak cough with whitish sputum, aversion to cold.
Tongue: Thin, white fur
Pulse: Superficial

Causes

External wind–cold factors block *qi*, for example cold air, draft, air conditioners, cool storage rooms.

Therapy

Expel wind–cold
Supplement lung
激 • LU-7 • TB-5 • GB-20 • LI-4

Avoid:
Raw, cool, and cold, as well as sour foods. *Thermal nature*: Hot for a short time, then warm, neutral.

Recommended:

Thermal nature	Hot for a short time; then warm, neutral
Organ network	Lung
Flavor	Acrid
Preparation methods	Boiled, steamed, fried
Vegetables	Green onions
Spices	Ginger, coriander, garlic, pepper, thyme, cinnamon

This syndrome can quickly change into wind–heat. If this happens, adapt therapy immediately!

Decoction of fresh ginger and green onions

■ Acute/Chronic Laryngitis

Dryness in Lung

Symptoms

Acute or chronic dry sore throat, hoarseness, dry cough, dry skin.
Tongue: Reddish
Pulse: Fast

Causes

External dryness enters the lung, vacuity of body fluids, condition shortly before lung *yin* vacuity develops, dry surroundings, heated air.

Therapy

Moisten lung
Replenish fluids
激 • LU-9 • KI-6 • LU-7
• LI-4 • LU-5 • SP-6

Avoid:
Acrid, sour, bitter foods with warm and hot thermal nature.

Recommended:

Thermal nature	Neutral and cool
Organ network	Spleen
Flavor	Sweet
Preparation methods	Boiled, steamed
Fruit	Pears, honeydew melons
Vegetables	Eggplant, button mushrooms
Nuts and seeds	Peanuts, pine nuts
Soy products	Soy milk

Banana with honey
(But not with phlegm conditions!)

Main Symptom: Frontal Sinusitis and Maxillary Sinusitis

Acute sinusitis	*Wind–heat invading the lung (feng re fan fei)*
Acute/chronic sinusitis	*Liver–gallbladder damp–heat (gan dan shi re)*
Recurrent sinusitis	*Lung qi vacuity, spleen qi vacuity* *Damp–heat in spleen (pi wei shi re)*

According to TCM:
Belongs to the "bi yuan" category, which literally means "nose pond," and refers to deep-source nasal congestion.

The main cause of sinusitis is repeated external attack of wind–heat or wind–cold (usually wind–heat). Sinusitis responds very well to acupuncture and herbal treatments, supported by dietary measures. Other causes of sinusitis are lung *qi* vacuity and spleen *qi* vacuity, both of which can be easily treated with nutritional therapy. Spleen *qi* vacuity, responsible for acute and chronic phlegm production, responds especially well to dietary measures.

■ Acute Sinusitis

Wind–Heat Invading the Lung (Feng Re Fan Fei)

Symptoms

Stuffy nose with white, mostly yellow secretion and crusting, partly blood-stained; headache, dry mouth, slight fever, aversion to wind.

Tongue: Thin, yellow fur
Pulse: Fast and superficial

Therapy

Expel wind–heat
Balance lung *qi*
激 • LI-20 • LI-4 • LI-11
• LU-10 • LU-7 • GB-20

Avoid:

Foods with sour flavor, for example lemon, or poultry (which pull pathogenic factors deeper into the body), foods with hot and warm thermal natures (too drying).

Recommended:

Thermal nature	Cool and cold
Organ network	Lung, spleen
Flavor	Mildly acrid (to expel pathogenic factors, but avoid producing heat), sweet (to moisten)
Preparation methods	Raw, boiled, steamed
To cool:	
Fruit	Mulberries, watermelons, pears, lemons, grapefruit
Vegetables	Dandelion, mung beans, radish, tomatoes
Grains	Wheat
Spices	Peppermint
For dryness:	
Fruit	Pears
Beverages	Pear juice, tomato juice, melon juice

Juice mix made from tomatoes and watermelon

For dryness:
Pear juice with honey

■ Acute/Chronic Sinusitis

Liver–Gallbladder Damp–Heat (Gan Dan Shi Re)

Symptoms

Stuffy nose, dryness, sticky and yellowish purulent secretion; foul-smelling, bitter taste in mouth; dry mouth and throat, headaches.

Tongue: Reddened on the side, yellow fur

Pulse: Fast, lateral

Causes

Combination of external wind–heat, excess heat and phlegm-producing foods (e.g., fatty and fatty foods, alcohol abuse); emotional strain, such as anger, rage, stress.

Therapy

Dispel liver–gallbladder damp–heat
Promote downbearing of lung *qi*
激 • LR-2 • LI-4 • GB-43
• LU-7 • GB-15

Avoid:

Thermally hot and warm foods, grilled food, acrid spices, alcoholic beverages, very fatty dishes, dairy products.

Recommended:

Thermal nature	Cool and cold
Organ network	Liver, gallbladder
Flavor	Bitter, salty, slightly sweet
Preparation methods	Raw, boiled, steamed
To disperse heat and remove dampness:	
Fish	Crayfish
Vegetables	Bamboo sprouts, mung beans, dandelion, celery root (celeriac)
Beverages	Green tea
To disperse heat:	
Vegetables	Bamboo shoots, Belgian endive hearts
Beverages	Gentian tea, green tea

Gentian tea, green tea

Pear juice with fresh lemon

■ Recurrent Sinusitis

Lung Qi Vacuity, Spleen Qi Vacuity

Symptoms

Stuffy nose, copious white–sticky or yellow–sticky viscous secretion, sometimes cough with watery or yellow–sticky sputum, loss of appetite, soft stools.

Tongue: Slightly red, white fur

Pulse: Weak and empty

Therapy

Supplement lung and spleen
激 • LU-9 • BL-13 • SP-2
• BL-20 • ST-36 • CV-6 • ST-40

Avoid:

Raw, cool, or cold foods, and bitter flavor.

Recommended:

Thermal nature	Neutral and warm
Organ network	Lung, spleen
Flavor	Slightly acrid, slightly sweet
Preparation methods	Boiled, steamed, fried
Meat	Duck
Fish	Carp
Fruit	Grapes
Vegetables	Cauliflower, carrots, onions
Grains	Oats, short-grain (glutinous) rice
Spices	Aniseed, ginger, garlic, rosemary, thyme
Nuts and seeds	Chestnuts, almonds, black sesame, sunflower seeds, walnuts
Other	Alcoholic beverages

Congee (see p. 117) made with rice, onions, and ginger

Avoid:

Raw, cold, and cool food, dairy products, excess sweets, excess meat.

Recommended:

(see also "Lung *Qi* Vacuity," p. 79)

Thermal nature	Neutral and warm
Organ network	Spleen, heart, lung
Flavor	Slightly sweet, slightly bitter, slightly acrid
Preparation methods	Boiled, fried, steamed
To transform phlegm:	
Fruit	Pears, cherries, apples
Vegetables	Leeks, radish
Grains	Millet
Spices	Ginger, garlic
To supplement spleen:	
Meat	Poultry, beef
Vegetables	Fennel, carrots
Grains	Oats, millet, rice
Spices	Aniseed, basil, ginger, coriander, thyme

■ Recurrent Sinusitis

Damp–Heat in Spleen (Pi Wei Shi Re)

Symptoms

Stuffy nose with copious yellow, foul-smelling secretion; pressure in head, sensation of heaviness in head and limbs; bitter, sticky taste in mouth.

Tongue: Yellow, sticky fur

Pulse: Fast, slippery

Causes

External dampness and heat, nutritional errors (irregular eating, too many acrid and fatty dishes).

Therapy

Supplement spleen
Remove heat and dampness

激 • SP-9 • LI-20 • CV-12 • BL-22 • LI-4

Avoid:

Raw, thermally hot and warm foods, excess sweets, dairy products, and alcoholic beverages.

Recommended:

Thermal nature	Cool, cold, and neutral
Organ network	Spleen
Flavor	Bitter
Preparation methods	Steamed, boiled
Vegetables	Artichokes, Belgian endive hearts, cucumbers, mung beans, celery
Beverages	Gentian tea, green tea, corn silk tea
Grains	Millet

Decoction of corn silk tea:
Steep about 50 g (1.5 oz) of corn silk in 1 L (four cups) of hot water; drink 1–2 L (four to eight cups) daily. Clears damp–heat and cools.

Decoction of corn silk tea and dandelion:
Steep about 50 g (1.5 oz) each of corn silk and dandelion in 1 L (four cups) of hot water; drink 1–2 L (four to eight cups) daily. Combining dandelion with corn silk increases the cooling and clearing effect of decoction.

Bronchial Asthma

Intrinsic (nonallergic) asthma	Phlegm–heat obstructing the lung (tan re zu fei)
Extrinsic (allergic) asthma	Wind–cold fettering the lung (feng han shu fei)
Chronic asthma	Lung qi vacuity and spleen qi vacuity Lung qi vacuity and kidney yang vacuity

According to TCM:
Shortness of breath (qi chuan bing) with or without accompanying sounds (gasping [xiao] due to phlegm) and with or without dyspnea (chuan).
Acute bronchial asthma is often caused by pathogenic factors such as wind–cold, heat, and phlegm. A chronic course or remission signifies an underlying lung, spleen, or kidney vacuity. These syndromes often overlap.
Consistent therapy combining acupuncture and herbs, supported by dietary measures and breathing exercise, for example qi gong, can produce good results.

■ Intrinsic (Nonallergic) Asthma

Phlegm–Heat Obstructing the Lung (Tan Re Zu Fei) (Acute Heat-Type Asthma)

Symptoms

Thick yellow viscous sputum that is difficult to cough up, frequent flat respiratory sounds, hasty breathing, thirst for cold drinks, fever.

Tongue: Yellow, sticky fur
Pulse: Fast, slippery

Causes

Inappropriate nutrition leading to spleen *qi* vacuity, external wind–heat factors.

Therapy

Transform phlegm
Cool heat inside lung
Stimulate *qi* coursing
激 • CV-17 • ST-40 • LU-5 • LU-6 • LI-4 • TB-5 • PC-6 • BL-13

Avoid:
Cold and overly acrid foods, excess sweet flavor, excess dairy products and meat (promotes production of phlegm), foods of a hot thermal nature (e.g., acrid spices).

Recommended:

Thermal nature	Neutral and cool, small amounts of cold
Organ network	Lung, spleen
Flavor	Mildly acrid, mildly sweet
Preparation methods	Raw, steamed, braised, boiled
Transformation of hot phlegm:	
Fruit	Pears, tangerines (peel), grapefruit (peel), lemons (peel preferably from organically grown fruit)
Vegetables	Bamboo sprouts, button or crimini/portobella mushrooms, dandelion, mung beans, radish, red marine algae (rhodophyta, red seaweed, or dulse)
Clear heat in lung:	
Fruit	Apples, pears
Vegetables	Seaweed, bamboo sprouts, watercress, Chinese (napa) cabbage, asparagus, radish, water chestnuts
Beverages	Peppermint tea
Grains	Pearl barley

Supplementing spleen:	
Meat	Poultry, beef
Vegetables	Fennel, carrots, sweet potatoes
Grains	Millet, rice
Spices	Aniseed

Radish juice, pear juice with fresh lemon

Extrinsic (Allergic) Asthma

Wind–Cold Fettering the Lung (Feng Han Shu Fei) (Acute Cold-Type Asthma)

Symptoms

Often copious whitish, watery sputum, gasping breathing sounds, aversion to cold, scratchy throat.

Tongue: White fur, damp
Pulse: Superficial

Causes

External pathogenic wind–cold binds *qi* in lungs, causing nondiffusion of lung *qi*; constitutional weakness.

Therapy

Expel of wind–cold
Transform phlegm
激 • LU-7 • BL-13 • ST-9 • CV-17 • ST-40

Avoid:

Raw, cool, and cold foods, foods that cause phlegm (dairy products, sweets, meat).

Recommended:

Thermal nature	Warm and neutral, possibly mildly hot
Organ network	Lung
Flavor	Acrid
Preparation methods	Boiled, steamed, fried
Vegetables	Green onions
Grains	Oats
Spices	Aniseed, ginger, coriander, thyme

Decoction of fresh ginger and green onions

Chronic Asthma

Lung Qi Vacuity and Spleen Qi Vacuity

Symptoms

Copious white sputum, fatigue, swollen extremities, lack of appetite, bloating in epigastric region after eating.

Tongue: Swollen, pale, white fur
Pulse: Weak

Causes

Persistent cough, weakened lung *qi*, constitutional weakness, lack of exercise, inappropriate diet that weakens the spleen.

Therapy

Supplement lung and spleen
激 • SP-3 • ST-36 • BL-20 • BL-21 • LU-9 • BL-13

Avoid:

Raw, cool, and cold foods, dairy products, excess sweet, excess meat.

Recommended:

(see also "Lung *Qi* Vacuity," p. 79)

Thermal nature	Neutral and warm
Flavor	Slightly acrid, slightly sweet
Organ network	Lung, spleen
Flavor	Mildly acrid, mildly sweet
Preparation methods	Boiled, steamed, fried
Meat	Duck
Fish	Carp
Fruit	Grapes
Vegetables	Cauliflower, carrots, onions
Grains	Oats, short-grain (glutinous) rice
Spices	Aniseed, ginger, garlic, rosemary, thyme
Nuts and seeds	Chestnuts, almonds, black sesame, sunflower seeds, walnuts
Other	Alcoholic beverages

To transform phlegm:

Fruit	Pears, cherries, apples
Vegetables	Leeks, radish
Grains	Millet
Spices	Ginger, garlic

To supplement spleen:

Meat	Poultry, beef
Vegetables	Fennel, carrots
Grains	Oats, millet, rice
Spices	Aniseed, basil, ginger, coriander, thyme

Congee (see p. 117) made with rice, onions, and ginger

Chronic Asthma

Lung Qi Vacuity and Kidney Yang Vacuity (Kidney is Unable to Receive Qi)

Symptoms

Cough, dyspnea, predominantly during inhalation (which is governed by the kidneys), dizziness, listlessness, clear urination during asthma attack, pain and weakness in knees and back.

Tongue: Moist, swollen, and pale
Pulse: Weak

Causes

Long-lasting chronic illnesses that weaken lung and kidney; inherited vacuity of the organ networks, excessive tension and strain. Because of kidney *qi* vacuity, the downbearing *qi* of the lungs can not be received, and accumulation of *qi* leads to a repletion condition, with fullness in the chest and dyspnea.

Therapy

Supplement and warm kidneys
Supplement lung

激 • KI-7 + Moxa • KI-3 + Moxa • BL-23 + Moxa • LU-7 • KI-6 • CV-17 • PC-6 • BL-13

Avoid:

Excess hot and acrid foods as well as raw, cold, and cool foods.

Recommended:

Thermal nature	Warm and a little hot, neutral
Organ network	Kidney, lung
Flavor	Salty, bitter
Preparation methods	Boiled, baked, fried, and grilled
To supplement and warm kidneys:	
Meat	Chicken, lamb, venison
Fish	Mussels, shrimp, oysters
Fruit	Raisins, grapes, cherries
Vegetables	Fennel
Grains	Oats, corn
Nuts and seeds	Chestnuts, walnuts
To supplement and downbear lung qi:	
Meat	Pork, duck
Fish	Mussels, pollack, carp, squid
Vegetables	Cauliflower, olives, onions
Other	Salted almonds

Gastrointestinal Disorders

Main Symptom: Diarrhea

Acute and chronic diarrhea	*Stomach qi and spleen qi vacuity* *Stomach yang and spleen yang vacuity* *Large intestine qi and yang vacuity*
Acute/chronic diarrhea	*Damp–cold encumbering the spleen (han shi kun pi)*
Infectious enteritis/traveler's diarrhea	*Damp–heat in spleen or large intestine*
Chronic morning diarrhea	*Spleen yang and kidney yang vacuity ("fifth watch diarrhea")*

According to TCM:
"Xie xie" means "flow discharge" and indicates soft and watery stools. This condition generally responds well to nutritional therapy, acupuncture, and possibly herbal therapy. Supplementing the center burner is also important.

General Nutritional Therapy

Rice, short-grain (glutinous) rice, millet, blueberries, button or crimini/portobella mushrooms, shredded apple; cooked, warm food.

Acute and Chronic Diarrhea

Stomach Qi and Spleen Qi Vacuity
Stomach Yang and Spleen Yang Vacuity
Large Intestine Qi and Yang Vacuity

Symptoms

Usually chronic diarrhea, watery and soft stools with undigested food particles, bloating after meals, improvement with pressure and warmth, flatulence after meals, physical weakness, lack of appetite.

Tongue: Pale, swollen with impressions
Pulse: Weak

Causes

Diet: Inappropriate diet that is too thermally cold, irregular meals.
General: Excessive worries, mental overexertion.

Therapy

Supplement spleen and stomach
激 • CV-12 • ST-36 • SP-2 • SP-3 • BL-20 • BL-21 • possibly Moxa!

Avoid:

Raw and thermally cool or cold foods (salads, fruit, fruit juices), dairy products, denatured foods, frozen food, canned food.

Recommended:

Boiled or steamed warming foods that build up spleen and stomach, combined with mildly acrid spices.

Thermal nature	Warm, neutral, possibly initially hot for a brief period
Organ network	Spleen, stomach
Flavor	Sweet–warm, sweet–neutral, possibly sweet–hot (briefly)
Meat	Poultry, beef
Fruit	Steamed apples, blueberries
Vegetables	Fennel, pureed carrots, button or crimini/portobella mushrooms, possibly some honey or brown sugar
Beverages	Fennel tea

Grains	Rolled oats, millet, rice, rice soup, short-grain (glutinous) rice with cinnamon and honey, slightly acrid rice dishes (warming effect)

Boiled millet porridge with cinnamon and raisins;

Rice cooked for a long time, with apple and cinnamon;

Carrot congee (see p. 117).

Acute/Chronic Diarrhea

Damp–Cold in Spleen or Large Intestine

Symptoms

Tendency to clear watery stool with undigested food particles, gurgling bowel sounds; improvement of stomach aches with warmth, worsening with pressure; aversion to cold, headaches, sensation of heaviness.

Tongue: White fur, moist, possibly slimy
Pulse: Slow, slippery

Causes

Diet: *Excess cold foods (e.g., ice tea) is a common cause of diarrhea in children during summer.*
General: Penetration of external cold and dampness (e.g., too much time spent in the swimming pool, wet clothes).

Therapy

Expel cold
Warm center burner
激 • ST-25 + Moxa
• ST-36 + Moxa • CV-12 + Moxa
• CV-6 + Moxa • SP-9

Avoid:
Raw, cold, and cool foods.

Recommended:

Thermal nature	Warm to hot, neutral
Organ network	Earth
Flavor	Sweet–warm, bitter–warm
Preparation methods	Boiled; steamed, possibly with alcohol; warming spices (e.g., ginger, pepper).
Vegetables	Fennel, carrots, sweet potatoes
Beverages	Fennel tea, spiced tea, coffee with cardamom
Grains	Oats, millet, rice with mildly acrid spices
Spices	Aniseed, chili, ginger, pepper, licorice, cinnamon

Ginger tea with cinnamon bark;

Coffee with cinnamon or cardamom;

Cinnamon rice with steamed apples.

Infectious Enteritis, Traveler's Diarrhea

Damp–Heat in Spleen or Large Intestine

Symptoms

Watery, soft, and foul smelling to stinking stools, tenesmus (constant feeling of the need to empty the bowel, accompanied by pain, cramping, and involuntary straining efforts), possibly bowel movement with blood, stomach aches that improve after bowel movement, hot burning sensation around anus, sparse dark urine, thirst.

Tongue: Thick, yellow fur, possibly slimy
Pulse: Fast and slippery

Causes

Diet: Inappropriate or spoiled foods.
General: Infections, penetration of external heat, and dampness into intestines.

Therapy

Dispel heat
Dry dampness
激 • ST-44 • LI-11 • BL-22 • CV-12
• ST-25 • SP-6 • SP-9 • PC-6

Avoid:
Acrid, warm, and hot foods.

Recommended:

Thermal nature	Cool, cold, and neutral
Organ network	Earth
Flavor	Sweet, bitter
Preparation methods	Raw, boiled, steamed
Fruit	Bananas, pears, honeydew melons, oranges, cranberries
Vegetables	Eggplant, bamboo sprouts, cucumbers, spinach, mung beans, dandelion
Beverages	Green tea, black tea, chamomile tea, wheat beer
Grains	Amaranth, corn
Spices	Yellow gentian
Dairy products	Yogurt
Soy products	Soy yogurt, tofu

Increase consumption of green or black tea and dried cranberries

Chronic Morning Diarrhea

Spleen Yang and Kidney Yang Vacuity

Symptoms

Chronic morning diarrhea! Stomach aches that improve with warmth, cold extremities, weakness in back and knees.

Tongue: Pale, impressions
Pulse: Weak, deep

Causes

General: Overwork, long-lasting illness, emotional stress, dissipated sex life, many births, exposure to cold.

Therapy

Warm kidneys
Supplement spleen
激 • CV-12 + Moxa • CV-4 + Moxa
• SP-6 + Moxa • BL-20 + Moxa
• ST-36 + Moxa • BL-23 + Moxa
• CV-6 + Moxa • SI-4 + Moxa • KI-7

Avoid:
Raw, cool, and cold foods.

Recommended:

Thermal nature	Warm to hot (briefly), neutral
Organ network	Kidney, spleen/pancreas
Flavor	Slightly salty, sweet
Preparation methods	Steamed, boiled, fried
Meat	Lamb, chicken
Fruit	Raisins, cherries
Vegetables	Fennel, leeks, carrots
Grains	Oats, short-grain (glutinous) rice, corn, millet
Spices	Aniseed, cinnamon, pepper, ginger
Nuts and seeds	Walnuts, chestnuts

Master Soup three times a week. Suggested ingredients: carrots, leek, beef, ginger, etc.

Main Symptom: Constipation

Constipation in elderly patients, postnatal constipation	*Qi vacuity or yang vacuity*
Constipation primarily in elderly patients	*Yin vacuity*
Constipation caused by stress or travel	*Liver qi stagnation*
	Chronic internal heat or heat in stomach and large intestine

According to TCM:
Infrequent bowel movements, abnormal stool shape, dry stools.

Responds very well to consistent dietary therapy, and also to combination of acupuncture and herbal therapy.

General Nutritional Therapy
Give preference to fruits and vegetables rich in fiber.

■ Constipation in Elderly Patients and Postnatal Constipation

Qi Vacuity or Yang Vacuity

Symptoms
Thinly formed, long stools; exertion and exhaustion after defecation, pale face, cold extremities. Seen especially in elderly patients and postpartum.
Tongue: Pale, swollen, moist
Pulse: Weak, deep

Causes
Qi vacuity or *yang* vacuity of the spleen, *yang* vacuity of the kidneys, exhaustion, aging, women after childbirth, after surgery, following long illnesses.

Therapy

Supplement *qi*
Supplement kidneys
Moisten intestine
激 • CV-4 + Moxa • CV-6 + Moxa
• SP-6 + Moxa • ST-36 + Moxa
• BL-20 • BL-21

Recommended:

Thermal nature	Warm and neutral
Organ network	Spleen, kidney, lung, large intestine
Flavor	Sweet, bitter, acrid
Preparation methods	Steamed, fried, boiled
Meat	Beef, poultry
Fruit	Dates, plums, cherries, peaches, apricots, figs
Vegetables	Fennel, radish, carrots, sweet potatoes
Beverages	Grape juice
Grains	Oats, rice, corn, soy
Spices	Aniseed, fresh ginger, garlic, marzipan, cinnamon
Nuts and seeds	Almonds, pine nuts, black sesame

Tip: Increase use of warming spices that promote digestion, such as pepper, coriander, capers, garlic.

■ Constipation Primarily in Elderly Patients

Yin Vacuity

Symptoms
Dry stool, dryness in mouth and throat (especially in the evening), night sweat, dizziness, ringing in the ears. Primarily seen in elderly patients.
Tongue: Red, chapped, without fur

Pulse: Superficial, empty

Causes

Aging (kidney *yin* vacuity), fluid deficiency in large intestine.

Therapy

Nourish yin
Supplement kidneys
Replenish body fluids
Moisten
激 • SP-6 • KI-6 • KI-3 • BL-23 • ST-36 • ST-25 (no moxibustion)

Avoid:
Bitter, acrid, and hot foods (too drying).

Recommended:

Thermal nature	Cool and neutral, for heat symptoms possibly slightly cold
Organ network	Spleen, lung, large intestine, kidney
Flavor	Sweet, salty
Preparation methods	Steamed, raw
Meat	Pork
Fruit	Bananas, pears, apples, apricots, plums
Vegetables	Seaweed, eggplant, Chinese (napa) cabbage, cucumbers, spinach, celery root (celeriac)
Grains	Wheat, barley, wheat germ
Spices	Salt
Nuts and seeds	Black sesame, peanuts
Soy products	Tofu

Walnuts with sesame
Walnuts with almonds and honey

Tip: Fresh fruits moisten and cool the digestive tract. Dried fruits concentrate sweetness, are mostly warming, absorb juices, moisten, and have a stronger laxative effect.

Constipation Caused by Stress or Travel

Liver Qi Stagnation

Symptoms

Sheeplike stool (small pellets), difficult bowel movement, belching, irritability. Usually caused by stress or travel.

Tongue: Slightly reddened sides
Pulse: Tense

Causes

Unresolved anger, stress, resentment.

Therapy

Loosen stagnation
Downbear *qi*
Moisten
激 • LR-3 • LI-4 • CV-12 • ST-36 • ST-25 • GB-34

Avoid:
Hot and fatty foods, acrid spices, fried or grilled foods.

Recommended:

Thermal nature	Neutral and cool, possibly a little cold
Organ network	Spleen
Phase	Wood
Flavor	Sour, possibly a little sweet, bitter–cool
Preparation methods	Raw, steamed, blanched
Fruit	Oranges, plums, grapefruit

Vegetables	Chinese (napa) cabbage, cucumbers, mung beans, spinach, tomatoes, celery stalks
Beverages	Bread juice, black tea, wheat beer, plum juice
Grains	Wheat, wheat germ
Nuts and seeds	Black sesame
Soy products	Tofu
Other	Yogurt, kefir, vinegar, apple cider

Wheat beer

Apple cider vinegar

Celery

Chronic Internal Heat, Heat in Stomach and Large Intestine

Symptoms

Dry, hard stools, infrequent bowel movements, thirst, dry mouth, pain and sensation of heat in abdomen.

Tongue: Red, dry yellow fur
Pulse: Fast

Causes

Too many acrid foods, stress.

Therapy

Clear heat
Moisten intestine
激 • LI-4 • LI-11 • TB-6 • ST-44
• ST-25 • SP-15 • SP-14 • ST-28

Avoid:

Hot foods and acrid spices.

Recommended:

Thermal nature	Cool and cold
Organ network	Liver, spleen, large intestine
Flavor	Sour, sweet
Preparation methods	Raw and steamed
Fruit	Apples, bananas, pears, kiwis, oranges, plums, grapefruit
Vegetables	Mung beans, spinach, rhubarb
Beverages	Pear juice, green tea, wheat beer
Grains	Wheat
Spices	Salt
Dairy products	Yogurt
Soy products	Tofu

Increase consumption of plum, pear, or orange juice.

Main Symptom: Epigastric Disorders

Acute and chronic gastritis, gastric ulcer, and duodenal ulcer	*Liver qi invading the stomach (gan qi fan wei)*
Gastric ulcer and duodenal ulcer	*Stomach fire (wei huo)*
	Stomach fire flaming upward (wei huo shang sheng)
	Liver fire flaming upward (gan huo shang yan)
Acute/chronic gastritis	*Stomach vacuity cold (wei qi xu han)* *Stomach qi vacuity*
Acute/chronic gastritis, gastric ulcer, and duodenal ulcer	*Stomach yin vacuity*

According to TCM:
Disorders of the epigastric region are summarized by the term "wei tong," which means "stomach pain," or "wei wan tong," which means "stomach duct pain." Both indicate stomach function disturbances.

Acute gastritis is more of a repletion syndrome, while chronic gastritis is more of a vacuity syndrome. Differential diagnosis is made by localization, duration, and type of symptoms.

General Nutritional Therapy

Reduce consumption of coffee, cigarettes, alcohol (high-proof), strongly spiced dishes (too warm/hot in thermal nature). Instead, several smaller (five) meals a day, prepared in a neutral or slightly warming way.

Tip: Generally recommended are white cabbage, white cabbage juice, carrots, dill, parsley, sage, basil.

■ Acute/Chronic Gastritis, Gastric Ulcer, and Duodenal Ulcer

Liver Qi Invading the Stomach (Gan Qi Fan Wei)

Symptoms

Attacks of cramplike pain in epigastric region, bloating, belching, nausea, retching, heartburn (stomach *qi* ascending counterflow, heat), bitter taste in mouth, irritability.

Tongue: Normal, sometimes white, thin fur; sometimes reddened sides

Pulse: Tense

Causes

One of the most common causes of acute and chronic epigastric pain is stagnation obstructing the upbearing of stomach *qi*. Other common causes are stress, anger, eating too fast; also liver *qi* stagnation, or ascending liver *yang* rooted in liver *yin* or kidney *yin* vacuity.

Therapy

Calm liver
Disperse *qi* stagnation
激 • LR-3 • GB-34 • PC-6
• CV-12 • LR-14 • ST-36

Avoid:
Acrid, hot, and fatty foods.

Recommended:

Thermal nature	Neutral, cool, and cold
Organ network	Liver, spleen, stomach
Flavor	Sour, sweet (possibly for a short time a little acrid and cool to remove stagnation)
Preparation method	Raw, steamed, boiled
Fish	Crab
Meat	Rabbit
Fruit	Apples
Vegetables	Brown seaweed, fennel, celery root (celeriac), celery stalks, (also white cabbage), spinach, water chestnuts
Beverages	Peppermint tea, black tea, wheat beer
Grains	Wheat
Dairy products	Yogurt

Avoid meat; seven-day diet of freshly ground, cooked grain porridge and black tea

■ Gastric Ulcer and Duodenal Ulcer

Stomach Fire (Wei Huo), Stomach Fire Flaming Upward (Wei Huo Shang Sheng), and Liver Fire Flaming Upward (Gan Huo Shang Yan)

Symptoms

Burning pain in epigastrium, bitter taste in mouth, heartburn, thirst, ravenous appetite, swollen and bleeding gums, nausea, vomiting, constipation, irritability, tendency towards outbursts of rage.

Tongue: Red, red sides, yellow fur

Pulse: Fast, full

Causes

Intense, protracted emotional burdens (lead to liver stagnation) that turn into heat/fire and attack the stomach. Anger, rage, inappropriate diet, excess acrid and hot foods, stress.

Therapy

Calm liver
Clear heat

激 • ST-44 • ST-21 • LR-13 • LR-14 • LR-2 • PC-6 • CV-12 • CV-13

Avoid:
Hot, acrid, and fatty foods.

Recommended:

Thermal nature	Cool and cold
Phase	Earth
Flavor	Sour, sweet
Preparation method	Raw, steamed, boiled
Fruit	Bananas, kiwis, watermelons
Vegetables	Seaweed, bamboo sprouts, Chinese (napa) cabbage, cucumbers, dandelion, mung beans, tomatoes, water chestnuts
Beverages	Gentian tea, green tea
Grains	Barley, wheat
Dairy products	Yogurt, cow's milk
Soy products	Tofu

■ Acute/Chronic Gastritis

Stomach Vacuity Cold (Wei Qi Xu Han) Stomach Qi Vacuity

Symptoms

Acute, dull pain in epigastrium, feeling of coldness, vomiting of clear liquids, improvement with warm beverages, cold extremities, lack of appetite.

Tongue: Pale; thick, white fur

Pulse: Deep, slow, weak

Causes

Inappropriate diet; penetration of external pathogenic cold, for example ice-cold beverages or cold foods, which burden stomach *qi*, lead to stagnation, and obstruct *qi* downbearing.

Therapy

Expel cold
Warm center burner
激 • CV-12 + Moxa • CV-6 + Moxa
• ST-36 + Moxa • SP-4
• BL-20 + Moxa • BL-21 + Moxa

Avoid:
Raw, cold, and cool foods.

Recommended:

Thermal nature	Warm, hot, and neutral
Organ network	Stomach, spleen/pancreas
Phase	Earth
Flavor	Sweet–warm, sweet–hot
Preparation methods	Boiled, steamed, fried (lightly)
Meat	Beef, chicken
Fish	Salmon, tuna
Fruit	Raisins, dates, papaya
Vegetables	Fennel, carrots, cabbage, potatoes, kohlrabi
Beverages	Fennel tea
Grains	Oats, millet, rice, corn
Spices	Increase use of warming spices, for example aniseed, ginseng, honey, ginger, cardamom, garlic, pepper, rosemary, cinnamon

Increase consumption of ginger tea, spiced tea, acridly spiced rice dishes, chicken dishes and beef dishes, warming and strengthening stocks and soups.

Acute/Chronic Gastritis, Gastric Ulcer, and Duodenal Ulcer
Stomach Yin Vacuity

Symptoms

Dull, burning pain in epigastric region, dry mouth, thirst, constipation, lack of appetite, sensation of heat in the afternoon.

Tongue: Red, chapped, no fur at center
Pulse: Fast

Causes

Diet: The most common causes are irregular and bad eating habits (too many late evening meals).
General: Protracted heat conditions, deficiency of body fluids, chronic stress, and overwork.

Therapy

Nourish stomach *yin*
Replenish fluids
激 • SP-6 • BL-20 • BL-21 • ST-36
• CV-12 • SP-3 • SP-9 • SP-4

Avoid:
Acrid, bitter, and hot foods, alcoholic beverages, acrid spices.

Recommended:

Thermal nature	For heat symptoms: cold; otherwise cool and neutral, a little warm
Organ network	Stomach, spleen/pancreas
Flavor	Sweet–neutral, sweet–cool
Preparation methods	Steamed, boiled, and baked in the oven
Cold foods:	
Fruit	Bananas, tomatoes, watermelons
Cool and neutral foods:	
Meat	Duck, fatty meat, pork
Fish	Bass, tuna

Fruit	Grapes, strawberries, apples
Vegetables	Carrots, eggplant, radish
Grains	Barley, millet, rice, wheat
Dairy products	Cheese, cow's milk, farmer's cheese, cottage cheese
Soy products	Tofu

Increase consumption of thermally neutral meat dishes that are high in fat, oven-baked casseroles, dairy products, white cabbage, and white cabbage juice.

Main Symptom: Nausea and Emesis (Vomiting)

Infectious emesis	*Cold evil invading the stomach (han xie fan wei)*
Acute/chronic emesis, motion sickness	*Stomach qi vacuity and cold*
Emesis following overeating	*Food stagnation in stomach*
Emesis caused by emotional strain	*Liver qi invading the stomach (gan qi fan wei)*
Chronic emesis	*Stomach yin vacuity*

According to TCM:
"Rebellious" stomach qi, or stomach qi flaming upward, is often caused by external pathogenic factors, especially cold, and also by emotional strain, constitutional weakness, and inappropriate diet. Differentiation between emesis with or without food particles.

Acute and chronic symptoms both respond very well to nutritional therapy, acupuncture, and herbs.

General Nutritional Therapy

Supplementing center burner, consumption of foods with downbearing effect.

Infectious Emesis

Cold Evil Invading the Stomach (Han Xie Fan Wei)

Symptoms

Sudden violent vomiting, often with food particles. Headache, aversion to cold, tension in epigastrium, shivering, fever.

Tongue: Thick, swollen; thick white fur
Pulse: Slow, deep

Causes

Inappropriate diet; penetration of external pathogenic cold, such as ice-cold drinks and cold foods, which burden stomach *qi*, lead to stagnation, and obstruct *qi* downbearing.

Therapy See below

Acute/Chronic Emesis

Stomach Qi Vacuity and Cold

Symptoms

Short, violent vomiting attacks with thin fluid (soft stools, lack of appetite, pale face, exhaustion).

Tongue: Pale, swollen; white fur
Pulse: Weak

Causes

Inappropriate diet, foods that are too cold, overwork, constitutional weakness.

Therapy

Expel cold
Warm center burner

- PC-6 • CV-12 + Moxa
- ST-36 + Moxa • SP-4 + Moxa
- ST-21 + Moxa

Avoid:

Raw, cool, and cold foods.

Recommended:

Thermal nature	Warm and hot
Organ network	Stomach, spleen/pancreas
Flavor	Sweet, acrid
Preparation methods	Boiled, steamed, fried
Vegetables	Fennel, carrots

Beverages	Tea made from fresh ginger; spiced teas with warming herbs, for example aniseed tea, fennel tea, cardamom, pepper, cinnamon; warming digestive liqueurs
Grains	Acridly seasoned rice or millet dishes, oats, corn
Spices	Aniseed, freshly grated ginger, fennel

Simmer a thumb-sized piece of ginger in 0.5 L (two cups) of water for 20 minutes; drink while warm.

Spiced teas

■ Emesis Following Overeating

Food Stagnation in Stomach

Symptoms

Nausea; sometimes vomiting of food particles, which brings relief; bloating in epigastrium, bad breath.

Tongue: Swollen; white, thick fur
Pulse: Full, slippery

Causes

Inappropriate diet (too many raw and cold foods, intake of cold beverages during meals, irregular meals, hasty eating, late evening meals).

Therapy

> **Disperse food stagnation**
> **Supplement center burner**
> 激 • PC-6 • ST-36 • CV-10 • ST-20 • ST-25 • ST-45 • LR-14

Avoid:

Excessive eating, main meals after 6 p.m., raw and cold foods

Recommended:

Thermal nature	Neutral and warm
Organ network	Stomach, spleen/pancreas
Flavor	Sweet, acrid (disperses stagnation)
Preparation method	Boiled, steamed, braised
Beverages	Aniseed schnapps, espresso, fennel tea, coffee, high-quality herbal liqueurs
Other	One to two teaspoons of vinegar

Keep high-quality herbal liqueurs at hand; nonalcoholic alternatives are fennel tea, freshly grated ginger, freshly brewed coffee with cinnamon and cardamom, espresso.

■ Emesis Caused by Emotional Strain

Liver Qi Invading the Stomach (Gan Qi Fan Wei)

Symptoms

Nausea and belching, sometimes with sour food particles; when anxious, pressure and bloating in epigastrium; frequent belching, irritability.

Tongue: Normal; sometimes white, thin fur; possibly reddened sides
Pulse: Tense

Causes

Mostly as a result of emotional strain. Stagnation of free coursing of stomach *qi*, for example due to anxiety, anger, frustration.

Therapy

> **Calm liver**
> **Disperse *qi* stagnation**
> 激 • LR-3 • GB-34 • PC-6 • CV-12 • LR-14 • ST-36

Avoid:
Acrid, hot, and fatty foods.

Recommended:

Thermal nature	Neutral, cool, and cold
Organ network	Liver, spleen, stomach
Flavor	Sour, sweet, (possibly for a short time a little acrid and cool to remove stagnation)
Preparation methods	Raw, steamed, boiled
Fish	Crab
Meat	Rabbit
Fruit	Apples, tangerines, grapefruit, pineapples, lemons
Vegetables	Brown seaweed, fennel, celery root (celeriac), spinach, water chestnuts, radish
Beverages	Peppermint tea, black tea, green tea, wheat beer
Grains	Wheat
Dairy products	Yogurt
Other	Vinegar, caraway seed

Abstain from eating meat; seven-day diet of freshly ground, cooked grain porridge and black tea.

■ Chronic Emesis

Stomach Yin Vacuity

Symptoms

Recurrent vomiting with small amounts of fluids, dry mouth, lack of appetite, overall weakness, exhaustion.

Tongue: Red, chapped; no fur in center
Pulse: Fast

Causes

Following long-term illnesses with loss of body fluids, overwork.

Therapy

Nourish stomach *ying*
Nourish fluids
Warm center burner
激 • PC-6 • ST-4 • ST-44
• ST-36 • SP-9 • KI-6

Avoid:
Acrid, bitter, and hot foods, alcoholic beverages, acrid spices.

Recommended:

Thermal nature	For heat symptoms: cold; otherwise cool and neutral, a little warm
Organ network	Stomach, spleen/pancreas
Flavor	Sweet
Preparation method	Steamed, boiled, baked in the oven
Cold foods:	
Fruit	Bananas, tomatoes, watermelons
Cool and neutral foods:	
Meat	Pork, duck, fatty meats
Fish	Tuna, bass
Fruit	Grapes
Vegetables	Carrots, potatoes
Grains	Millet, rice, barley, corn
Dairy products	Cow's milk, cheese, farmer's cheese, cottage cheese
Soy products	Tofu

Increase consumption of fatty, thermally neutral meat dishes, casseroles baked in the oven, and dairy products.
Subsequently: Supplement center burner.

■ Inflammatory Gastrointestinal Disorders, Crohn Disease, Ulcerative Colitis

According to TCM:
Differential diagnosis is made according to symptoms, for example diarrhea, blood in stool, sloppy stools.

Good results can be achieved by combining conventional allopathic medicine, Chinese dietetics, acupuncture, and herbal therapy.

In severe cases, conventional medicine and TCM should work hand in hand at the beginning. As soon as the TCM treatment starts showing good results, the intake of allopathic medications can be reduced and finally stopped. Such treatments should only be undertaken by an experienced TCM practitioner.

Therapy
Determined by the following TCM syndromes, which usually occur simultaneously.

Stomach qi and spleen qi vacuity

Liver qi invading the stomach and spleen (gan qi fan wei, gan qi fan pi)

Large intestinal damp–heat (da chang shi re)

Kidney yang vacuity

Spleen yang vacuity

■ Stomach *Qi* and Spleen *Qi* Vacuity

Symptoms
Loose, frequent, slimy and bloody stools; uncomfortable feeling of pressure in lower abdominal region, lack of appetite, weight loss, overall weakness, pale face.
Tongue: Pale, swollen
Pulse: Weak

Causes
Weak spleen *qi* no longer able to retain blood; inappropriate diet, weakened *qi* due to liver attack brought on by unresolved emotional burdens.

Therapy

Supplement stomach and spleen
激 • CV-12 • ST-36 • BL-20 • BL-21 • SP-3 • ST-25 • SP-10 • ST-25 • ST-27 • CV-66 • possibly Moxa

Avoid:
Raw, cool, and cold foods.

Recommended:

Thermal nature	Neutral and warm
Organ network	Stomach, spleen/pancreas
Flavor	Sweet
Preparation methods	Boiled, steamed
Meat	Chicken, beef
Vegetables	Fennel, sweet potatoes
Beverages	Aniseed tea, fennel tea
Grains	Millet, oats, rice
Spices	Honey

Consistent rice and millet diet with warming vegetables and lightly warming spices (especially cooked carrots, potatoes, coriander for stomach cold); fennel tea.

■ Liver *Qi* Invading the Stomach and Spleen
(Gan Qi Fan Wei, Gan Qi Fan Pi)

Symptoms
Cramplike pain attacks in epigastric region, bloating, belching, nausea, retching, heartburn (stomach *qi* flaming upward, heat), bitter taste in mouth, irritability.
Tongue: Normal; possibly white, thin fur; possibly reddened sides
Pulse: Tense

Causes

One of the most frequent causes of acute and chronic epigastric pain is stagnation obstructing stomach *qi*. Other common causes are stress, anger, hasty eating, as well as liver *qi* stagnation or ascending liver *yang*, rooted in liver *yin* vacuity or kidney *yin* vacuity.

Large Intestinal Damp–Heat
(Da Chang Shi Re)

Symptoms

Loose, slimy, purulent stools, sometimes mixed with blood; pain in hypochondrium (upper lateral region of the abdomen, marked by the lower ribs), subfebrile temperatures in the afternoon, thirst.

Tongue: Thick; firm fur, perhaps slimy
Pulse: Fast, slippery

Causes

Weak spleen *qi* can no longer transform fluids; inappropriate diet (hot, acrid, and fatty dishes) and emotional stress lead to heat symptoms.

Therapy

Dispel heat
Drain dampness
激 • ST-44 • LI-11 • BL-22 • CV-12
• ST-25 • SP-6 • SP-9 • PC-6

Avoid:
Acrid, warm, and hot foods.

Recommended:

Thermal nature	Cool, cold and neutral
Phase	Earth
Flavor	Sweet, bitter
Preparation methods	Raw, boiled, steamed
Fruit	Bananas, pears, honeydew melons, oranges
Vegetables	Eggplant, bamboo sprouts, cucumbers, spinach
Beverages	Chamomile tea, black tea, green tea, wheat beer
Spices	Yellow gentian
Dairy products	Yogurt
Soy products	Tofu

Increase intake of green or black tea.

Kidney *Yang* Vacuity

According to TCM:
Source of different vacuity syndromes, primarily vacuity in center burner (stomach qi and spleen qi vacuity or spleen yang vacuity).

Symptoms

Morning diarrhea, stomach aches that get better with warmth, cold extremities, weakness in back and knees.

Tongue: Pale with impression
Pulse: Weak, deep

Causes

Overwork, protracted illness, emotional stress, dissipated sex life, many births, exposure to cold.

Therapy

Warm kidney *yang*
激 • KI-3 • KI-7 • BL-23
• Moxa

Avoid:
Raw, cool, and cold foods.

Recommended:

Thermal nature	Warm to hot (briefly), neutral
Organ network	Kidney, spleen/pancreas
Flavor	Slightly salty, sweet
Preparation methods	Steamed, boiled, fried
Meat	Lamb, venison, beef, chicken
Fruit	Raisins, cherries, grapes
Vegetables	Fennel, leeks
Grains	Oats, short-grain (glutinous) rice, corn
Spices	Aniseed, cinnamon, rosemary
Nuts and seeds	Walnuts, chestnuts, black sesame

Master Soup with ingredients that supplement the kidney organ network, such as carrots, leek, lamb.

Spleen *Yang* Vacuity

Symptoms
Loss of appetite, hiccoughs, nausea, retching, soft stools, diarrhea. With *yang* vacuity: Cold extremities, fatigue, exhaustion.
Tongue: Pale, swollen with impression
Pulse: Weak

Causes
Inappropriate diet, overexertion, irregular intake of food, long, draining illnesses.

Therapy

Supplement stomach and spleen
激 • CV-12 • ST-36 • SP-6
• BL-20 • BL-21

Avoid:
Raw and thermally cool or cold foods (e.g., salads, fruit, fruit juices), dairy products, denatured foods, frozen foods, canned foods.

Recommended:
Warming foods that supplement stomach and spleen, seasoned with slightly warming spices.

Thermal nature	Neutral, warm, hot
Flavor	Sweet–warm, sweet–neutral, possibly sweet–hot (briefly)
Organ network	Stomach, spleen/pancreas
Preparation methods	Boiled, steamed
Meat	Chicken, lamb, beef
Fruit	Steamed apples, blueberries
Vegetables	Button or crimini/portobella mushrooms, fennel, pureed carrots, leeks, sweet potatoes
Beverages	Fennel tea
Grains	Oats, millet, rice, rice soup, rice dishes lightly seasoned with warming spices (see below, warming effect), short-grain (glutinous) rice with cinnamon and honey
Spices	Aniseed, honey, ginger, coriander, garlic, caraway seed, brown sugar

Cooked millet porridge with cinnamon and raisins.

Main Symptom: Meteorism (Abdominal Distension)

"Acute" meteorism	*Qi stagnation with food retention in stomach and spleen*
"Recurrent" meteorism	*Stomach qi vacuity, spleen qi vacuity,* stomach or spleen yang vacuity

According to TCM:
"Du zi zhang," which means belly distention, or "gu chang/fu zhang," which means drum/abdominal distention (Wiseman).

Differential diagnosis according to repletion and vacuity conditions, primarily caused by dysfunction of spleen and stomach. Responds very well to nutritional therapy.

General Nutritional Therapy

Prepare dishes using warming spices, such as caraway seed, coriander, chili, and vinegar.

Thermal nature	Warm
Organ network	Stomach, spleen
Flavor	Sweet, acrid
Preparation methods	Steamed, boiled
Vegetables	Fennel, carrots, leeks
Beverages	Fennel tea, caraway seed tea, warming, acrid herbal liqueurs
Spices	Aniseed, garlic, coriander, chili, star anise, pepper

Increase use of warming spices, improve eating habits, increase consumption of spiced teas.

"Acute" Meteorism

Qi Stagnation with Food Retention in Stomach and Spleen

Symptoms

Loud flatulence sounds, bloating, complaints worsen with pressure, possibly nausea and vomiting, bad breath, possibly constipation.

Tongue: Thick yellow fur
Pulse: Fast, slippery

Causes

Irregular food intake, inappropriate diet

Therapy

Disperse *qi* stagnation
激 • CV-12 • ST-25 • ST-36
• CV-6 • LI-4

Avoid:
Raw, cool, and cold foods.

Recommended:
Give preference to slightly acrid foods and spices with digestive effect.

"Recurrent" Meteorism

Stomach Qi and Spleen Qi Vacuity
Stomach or Spleen Yang Vacuity

Symptoms

Quiet flatulence sounds, bloating improves with pressure and warmth, lack of appetite, fatigue, soft stools, light urine.

Tongue: Pale; white fur
Pulse: Weak

Causes

Inappropriate diet, constitutional weakness, overwork

Therapy

Supplement stomach and spleen
激 • ST-36 + Moxa • CV-4 + Moxa
• SP-3 + Moxa • ST-25

Avoid:
Raw, cold, and cool foods.

Recommended:

Thermal nature	Neutral, warm, and hot
Organ network	Stomach, spleen, pancreas
Flavor	Sweet, acrid
Preparation	Boiled, steamed, fried
Vegetables	Fennel, cooked carrots
Beverages	Aniseed tea, warming herbal liqueurs
Grains	Oats, millet, rice
Spices	Aniseed, ginger, garlic, coriander, caraway seed

Warming spiced teas, warming spices with slightly acrid flavor, acridly seasoned dishes, for example, millet and rice casseroles. For children, especially fennel tea, cooked carrots, improvement of eating habits, regular meals.

Main Symptom: Hiccough, Singult (Sighing, Sobbing)

Cold evil invading the stomach (han xie fan wei)

According to TCM:
"Rebellious" or counterflow stomach qi; retching primarily due to cold in the stomach. Responds well to acupuncture and nutritional therapy.

■ Cold Evil Invading the Stomach *(Han Xie Fan Wei)*

Symptoms

Heavy, deep belching which improves with heat; lack of appetite, exhaustion.

Tongue: Pale; white fur
Pulse: Slow

Causes

Inappropriate diet, excess of raw and cold foods, irregular eating habits, constitutional *qi* vacuity.

Therapy

Downbear stomach *qi*
Warm stomach
激 • CV-12 • BL-17 • PC-6
• CV-12 • ST-36 • ST-21

Recommended:

Thermal nature	Neutral and warming
Organ network	Stomach, spleen/pancreas
Flavor	Sweet
Direction	Downbearing
Preparation methods	Steamed, boiled, fried
Beverages	Ginger juice
Spices	Aniseed, fennel, freshly grated ginger, coriander

Obesity/Losing Weight

Main Symptom: Overweight

Overweight	*Spleen qi or spleen yang vacuity (pi qi xu, pi yang xu)*
	Retention of dampness and/or phlegm
	Blazing stomach fire with phlegm
	Liver qi stagnation/liver qi invading the stomach/spleen (gan qi fan wei, gan qi fan pi)
	Kidney yang vacuity (shen yang xu)

According to TCM:
The main cause is a disturbance and weakness in spleen function, accompanied by the formation of dampness and phlegm retention. It is not uncommon for liver qi stagnation, by affecting the control cycle, to cause "depression of the inner center" and blockage and weakness of the spleen. In ancient China, being overweight was long regarded as a sign of prosperity and wealth, hence we do not find any direct classical recommendations for the treatment of obesity, since this was not a desirable goal. Nevertheless, the differentiated approaches of TCM in the diagnosis of individual syndromes and in the individual application of Chinese dietetics are still ideal for the treatment of "modern" health problems.

The causes of obesity are generally multilayered by nature. For effective permanent weight loss, a change in lifestyle is always important. Primarily, this includes adjustments in diet and nutrition, an attentive attitude towards nutrition, regular physical activity, and, if necessary, complementary psychotherapeutic measures.

In this context, acupuncture can have an excellent supporting and harmonizing effect as a complementary measure and can be used to reduce the appetite, but the most important factor is still a change in diet.

General Nutritional Therapy

As the first step, patients should direct their attention to their daily eating habits. We highly recommend keeping an eating journal, that is, recording in detail for at least a week how and what you eat throughout the day; which preferences exist; how much dairy products, raw foods, fruit, etc., you consume; personal eating behavior (in quiet, in front of the TV, gulping it down or chewing it slowly). You should also observe how much you eat "in between" and what these snacks consist of. These records are then analyzed and interpreted by the therapist, and a therapy of syndrome balance follows. We offer the following general tips: Regular meal times are important. It is best to eat breakfast between 7 and 11 a.m. (the best time for spleen and stomach functions), lunch between 12 and 2 p.m., and dinner between 5 and 8 p.m.

Recommended:

You should eat at least three meals in the course of the day:

- A good breakfast that has a warming and supporting effect on the spleen, such as millet gruel, oats, or amaranth muesli, etc. Avoid the popular but cooling fruit juices (except under certain circumstances in the summer) as well as cooling and phlegm-producing dairy products. These weaken the spleen in the morning and, due to the resulting dampness, block spleen *qi*.

- Depending on constitution, lunch should be the main meal of the day.
- In the afternoon a light snack may be eaten.
- Dinner should not be too sumptuous and should not be consumed too late. The best time is between 6 and 8 p.m. Later meals coincide with the weak time of the spleen and are especially prone to causing weight gain.
- Before lunch or dinner, a light snack may be consumed.

Cooked and fermented foods are preferable, if necessary well seasoned, especially in the winter. In the summer, raw foods may be eaten in greater quantities. Chew every bite well; 10–15 times would be best.

During meals, drink only small amounts because excess fluid consumption weakens the *qi* of the stomach. The greatest consumption of fluids should occur between meals. Depending on body size and time of the year, between 1.5 and 3 L.

For breakfast, energetically warming drinks are recommended, e.g., fennel tea (especially for children), spice teas, ginger tea, and black tea where appropriate. In the summer, also green tea. Under all circumstances, avoid strongly cooling drinks like orange juice.

As a lunch and dinner drink, we recommend water, or when appropriate also light alcoholic drinks. After a good meal, you may also enjoy a high-proof digestif to release a *qi* blockage and potential accumulation of fluids. Before meals, an alcoholic aperitif can warm and move spleen and stomach *qi*.

In patients with severe obesity, we initially recommend a radical change in diet, accompanied by one to two acupuncture treatments per week. At the start, a complete fast or a rotation diet, lasting between 1 and 3 weeks, can be remarkably effective. Radical weight loss is not necessarily desirable, but rather a weight reduction of 2–6 kg per month. Sufficient fluid intake, preferably water, is important. At this stage, meat products should be reduced drastically or, better yet, avoided altogether; the same holds true for sugar, alcohol, and other stimulants. Reducing dairy products, yogurt, cheese, raw foods, and fruit (tropical fruit) is also desirable.

In the reduction phase, you must be careful not to weaken kidney *qi* too much. From this perspective, warming and tonifying foods are recommended (spice tea, ginger).

In the course of these radical dietary restrictions and changes, it is important to develop gradually a permanent awareness for a new and different way of eating. Of course, this includes as many fresh, high-quality, natural foods, as "rich in *qi*" as possible. A regular rhythm for meals should be maintained as well, preferably in a comfortable environment without pressure or distraction. It is important to perceive eating as a positive experience and to remember that it is the most important factor for regenerating and strengthening *qi* and bodily fluids. We advise against irregular, sporadic food intake or sumptuous late meals because they invariably lead to weight gain.

After the food-restricted phase, tonifying the spleen is indispensable because this is the key to a stable body weight. The spleen must always be "fed" and supported; this is the only way that we can avoid repeated weight gain.

Avoid:
Too many dairy products, excessive consumption of meat and alcohol, excessive fat consumption, excessive consumption of sweets, irregular food intake, eating too quickly, foods of inferior quality. Skipping breakfast and, after lunch with only a snack in between, dinner as the main meal of the day.

Prognosis

The condition of obesity can be treated extremely well with the knowledge and methods of TCM. Experience shows that a changed diet in conjunction with acupuncture leads to a weight loss of up to 15 kg in 3–6 months. Daily eating habits ("cultivating the inner center") must be developed over time as described above if this result is to be permanent.

Therapy

Main points

激 • ST-36 • ST-34 • SP-4
• SP-10 • LI-11 • LI-4

For excessive appetite

激 • ST-44

For obstipation

激 • ST-25 • TB-5

To conduct dampness

激 • SP-9

Ear acupuncture

激 In addition to generally differentiated body acupuncture, ear acupuncture with permanent needles is an excellent therapeutic tool.
Points of the abdominal zone: ear points 55 *shen men*, 51 autonomous nervous system, 29 cushion, antiaggression point, antidepression point

■ Overweight

Spleen Qi or Spleen Yang Vacuity

Symptoms

Obesity with slack fat tissue, few muscles, patient eats little, easily becomes tired and exhausted, little thirst, almost no desire to drink, sloppy stools.
Tongue: Pale, swollen with dental impressions
Pulse: Faint, weak

Causes

Mostly wrong eating habits, mental strain, climatic conditions, and chronic illnesses. In addition, a constitutional weakness of the digestive organs can also lie at the root of spleen *qi* vacuity.

Therapy

Supplement spleen *qi* and spleen *yang*

激 • SP-3 • SP-2 • BL-20 • BL-21 • ST-36
• CV-12 + Moxa

Avoid:

Foods with a cold or cooling thermal nature, cold or iced drinks; excessive consumption of raw foods such as salads and fruit; dairy products such as cottage cheese, farmer's cheese, cheese, milk, sour milk products; tofu; thermally cold drinks like black or green tea, wheat beer, mineral water, thermally cold fruit juices like orange juice; tomatoes, cucumbers, tropical fruits, oranges, lemons, bananas, kiwis, pineapple, watermelon; an excess of spicy and sweet flavors (refined sugar)!

Recommended:

Fish	Warming types of fish such as salmon, trout, tuna, shellfish
Meat	Beef (beef bouillon), chicken (chicken broth), lamb
Fruit	Sweet cherries, plums, peaches, sweet apples, jujubes, apricots, dates, figs, red grapes, dried fruit (raisins, figs, prunes, dates, apricots)
Vegetables	Warming vegetables like fennel, carrots, sweet potatoes, pumpkin, sautéed onions, cabbage
Beverages	Fennel tea, spice tea with cinnamon, mead, liqueurs, malt beer, licorice tea, red grape juice, corn silk tea
Grains	Millet, oats, sweet rice, rice, buckwheat, amaranth, polenta
Spices	Cayenne pepper, ginger, cinnamon, cardamom, nutmeg, vanilla, star anise, anise, fennel seed, but also spices of the fire phase like coriander, oregano, rosemary, thyme
Sweeteners	Honey, raisins, barley malt, maple syrup, cane sugar
Nuts and seeds	Pine nuts, pistachios, peanuts, hazelnuts, coconuts, sesame

Tip: Generally recommended are foods with the sweet–warm and sweet–hot flavors for strengthening the earth phase; also neutral foods. Regular food intake is important: at least one warm meal a day!

Retention of Dampness and Phlegm

Symptoms

Hypertension, feeling of heaviness in head and extremities; slowed, "dragging" movement; feeling of pressure in chest, dizziness, fatigue, excess weight.

Tongue: Pale; thick white slimy fur
Pulse: Slippery

Causes

Primarily due to inappropriate diet (e.g., excess fatty meat, dairy products, sweets), weakening of spleen, obesity, stress, and overexhaustion.

Therapy

Strengthen the spleen
Transform dampness and phlegm
Strengthen the kidneys

激 • ST-40 • CV-22 • PC-6 • SP-3 • BL-20 • BL-21 • KI-7 • BL-23

Avoid:

Strongly phlegm-producing foods, especially dairy products, bananas, very fatty and oily foods, junk food, excess of sweets, drinks that contain sugar. Excess of *yin* foods (note the time of year and climate!): raw foods, salads, and fruits with a cool and cold nature, citrus fruit juices. Avoid frozen foods and preparing/heating food in the microwave. Beware: when consumed in excess, meat easily produces phlegm, especially pork; alcohol has a similar effect.

Recommended:

To strengthen the spleen:

All foods that strengthen the spleen, to avoid further formation of dampness and phlegm (see spleen–pancreas *qi* vacuity and *yang* vacuity). Millet in particular supplements and warms the spleen while at the same time having a drying effect on disproportionate moistness in the body.

To transform dampness and heat phlegm:

Thermal nature	Cool
Flavor	Bitter, salty, occasionally also sweet
Fruit	Pears
Vegetables	Chicory, dandelion, mung beans, radishes, red marine algae (dulse), seaweed
Spices	Salt
Soy products	Soy milk

To transform dampness and cold phlegm (whitish, clear, thin):

Thermal nature	Warm
Flavor	Bitter, spicy
Vegetables	Chinese leeks
Spices	Fresh ginger (in moderation), garlic, cardamom

Tip: For phlegm blocking the flow of *qi* in the channels: moderately spicy taste flavor can disperse the stagnation, e.g., pungent spices like pepper, garlic, ginger.

Porridge of short-grain rice or warm porridge in the morning (see p. 115).

Blazing Stomach Fire with Phlegm (Heat Congestion in the Stomach)

Symptoms

Overweight with strong musculature, fat belly; patient eats a lot and with gusto (strong feeling of hunger); frequent foul bad breath; dry stool, frequent constipation; very thirsty, concentrated urine; tendency to hypertonicity.

Tongue: Red, thick/yellow fur

Pulse: Rapid, replete, forceful

Causes

Strong persistent emotional strain causes liver stagnation that transforms into fire and invades the stomach. Alternatively, anger, rage, malnourishment, excessive consumption of spicy and hot foods, stress. This condition is a repletion heat syndrome of the stomach in which the fluids have dried up.

Therapy

Cool and expel stomach heat; downbear stomach *qi*

激 • ST-44 • ST-45 • CV-12 • PC-6 • CV-10 • CV-13

Avoid:

Hot, spicy, fatty, and strongly seasoned foods, hot spices, high-proof alcohol, coffee, red wine, smoking.

Recommended:

Thermal nature	Cool and cold
Flavor	Sour–cold, sour–cool, sweet–cold, sweet–cool, bitter–cool
Preparation methods	Cooling
Fruit	Bananas, watermelon, kiwis
Vegetables	Tomatoes, bamboo sprouts, dandelion, celery root (celeriac), water chestnuts, mung beans, Chinese (napa) cabbage, seaweed, cucumbers
Beverages	Gentian tea, green tea
Grains	Wheat, barley
Dairy products	Yogurt
Soy products	Tofu

Liver Qi Stagnation, Liver Qi Invading the Stomach/Spleen

Symptoms

Feeling of fullness, belching, nausea, heartburn (rebellious stomach *qi*, heat), bitter taste in the mouth, irritability. Occasionally spasmodic cramp-like pain in the upper abdomen.

Tongue: Normal, occasionally thin white fur or reddish sides

Pulse: Tense

Causes

Blockages prevent the upbearing of stomach *qi* and spleen function. Common causes are stress, anger, hurried eating. Liver *qi* stagnation or ascendant liver *yang* are commonly found at the root of liver *yin* or kidney *yin* vacuity.

Therapy

Calm the liver, disperse *qi* stagnation

激 • LR-3 • LI-4 • PC-6 • CV-12 • LR-14 • ST-36

Avoid:
Spicy, hot, and fatty foods, meat, high-proof alcohol.

Recommended:

Thermal nature	Neutral, cool, and cold
Organ network/flavor	Liver and sour; spleen/stomach and sweet (on occasion slightly spicy and cool as needed to disperse stagnation)
Preparation method	Raw, steamed, boiled
Fruit	Plums
Vegetables	Radishes, celery
Beverages	Peppermint tea
Spices	Ginger, pepper, garlic, coriander, chili

Abstain from eating meat; 7-day diet of freshly ground, cooked grain porridge and black tea.

Kidney Yang Vacuity (Shen Yang Xu)

Symptoms

Accumulation of fat, especially on the abdomen and buttocks, large soft thighs, patient eats normally, frequent urination, feeling cold, sloppy stool, weakness and pain in the back and lower body; in men: frequently impotence; in women: dysmenorrhea, amenorrhea.

Tongue: Pale
Pulse: Faint, deep

Causes

In addition to constitutional *yang* vacuity, the causes lie primarily in lifestyle and nutrition. Hence, stress, overwork, lack of sleep, excessive sexual activity, births too close together, and an excess of negative emotions play a large role. An excess of thermally cold foods, *yin* products, irregular food intake, iced drinks, and eating canned food are additional factors. Exposure to cold also contributes.

Therapy

Strengthen and warm kidney *yang* and the *ming men*

激 • KI-7 • GV-4 • CV-4 • CV-6 • BL-23 + Moxa

Strengthen the *ming men*

激 • GV-4 + Moxa

Avoid:
All thermally cool or cold foods, frozen foods, raw foods, salads, sour milk products, thermally cold fruit and drinks. In addition, refined sugar and alcohol have a strong weakening effect on kidney *qi*.

Recommended:

Thermal nature	Neutral, warm, moderately hot
Flavor	Hot–salty, warm–salty, neutral–salty
Meat	Game meat (especially venison), pigeon, duck, pork
Fish	Trout, lobster, salmon, smoked fish
Vegetables	Fennel, cabbage, leeks, horseradish, root vegetables, onions
Grains	Millet, rice, sweet rice, buckwheat, oats
Spices	Ginger, garlic, black pepper, cinnamon
Nuts and seeds	Chestnuts, black sesame, sunflower seeds, roasted walnuts

Tip: **A good breakfast is important: warm grain porridge, millet, and oats. At least two warm meals a day. Use pungent *yang* spices and Master Soup (see p. 33) with warming kinds of meat, vegetables.**

Physical and/or Emotional Fatigue

Main Symptoms: Fatigue, Exhaustion, Burnout

Short-term fatigue, feebleness	*Spleen qi vacuity (pi qi xu)*
Short-term fatigue, feebleness	*Spleen yang vacuity (pi yang xu)*
Short-term fatigue, feebleness, blockage	*Liver qi stagnation (gan qi yu jie)*
Longer-term fatigue, exhaustion	*Kidney yang vacuity (shen yang xu)*
Longer-term fatigue, exhaustion, burnout	*Kidney yin vacuity (shen yin xu)*
Longer-term fatigue, exhaustion, burnout	*Liver yin vacuity (gan yin xu)*
Longer-term fatigue, exhaustion, burnout	*Liver blood vacuity (gan xue xu)*
Longer-term fatigue, exhaustion, burnout	*Blood vacuity—lack of blood (xue xu)*

According to TCM:
While these terms are unknown as such in TCM, they are rapidly becoming increasingly prevalent in the Western as well as presumably in the Eastern world. TCM offers excellent options for treating these problems—most significantly by means of dietetic measures and Chinese herbal therapy.

Etiology

The causes are manifold. Under a combination of excess physical and psychological strain, a therapeutic analysis often reveals a lack of attention to the patient's own physical energy and resources. It is obviously important in this situation to search for possible causes in biomedical terms as well (from thyroid dysfunction to tumors).

The syndromes of recurring fatigue, exhaustion, and burnout blend seamlessly into each other. The same is true for the Chinese patterns: *qi* stagnation is followed by *qi* vacuity, then *yang* vacuity. If the condition is compounded by heat, such as from stress or alcohol, the *yin* of the viscera is damaged and exhausted.

General symptoms are fatigue, lack of appetite, feebleness, sleeping disorders, a need for longer periods of regeneration, sensation of cold in the body, listlessness, exhaustion, depressed mood.

Therapy addresses several levels. For dispersing liver *qi* stagnation, acupuncture and Chinese herbal therapy are ideal tools. In the case of other syndromes, especially for building *yin*, blood, and fluids, Chinese dietetics is most important. These disorders respond well to treatment in combination with acupuncture and Chinese herbal therapy.

Prognosis

Depending on the severity of the condition, from mild fatigue to chronic fatigue, exhaustion, or burnout, therapeutic success results within 1–6 months. In classic burnout syndrome (kidney *yin* vacuity/liver *yin* vacuity), therapy may well require 1–2 years. It is common for dietary measures to show results only after 4–8 weeks, even if implemented consistently, but they build up consistently afterwards. When combined with consistent herbal therapy, the length of treatment can usually be shortened by 30%. It is important that the patient regularly integrates all measures into his or her life and practices good "vital *qi* cultivation." This includes:

- Regular eating (3–5 meals a day)
- High-quality nutrition according to the rules of TCM
- Sufficient sleep
- Regular physical exercise
- Relaxation techniques (*qi gong, tai chi*, yoga, meditation)

Short-term Fatigue, Feebleness

Spleen Qi Vacuity (Pi Qi Xu)

Symptoms

Chronic fatigue, general feebleness, recurring susceptibility to infections, lack of appetite, weak forceless limbs, craving sweets, pale sallow complexion, soft sloppy stools (occasionally chronic diarrhea).

Tongue: Pale, swollen, puffy, moist
Pulse: Vacuous, weak, possibly slow

Causes

One of the most common syndromes in clinical practice, it leads patients into the doctor's office with a variety of symptoms and can be caused by wrong eating habits, mental strain, climatic conditions, and chronic illnesses. In addition, a constitutional weakness of the digestive organs can also lie at the root of spleen *qi* vacuity.

Therapy

Supplement spleen *qi*
激 • SP-3 • SP-2 • BL-20 • BL-21 • ST-36 • CV-12 + Moxa

Avoid:

Foods with *yin* characteristics, with cold or cooling thermal nature, cold or iced drinks, excessive consumption of raw foods such as salads and fruit, dairy products such as farmer's cheese, cottage cheese, cheese, milk, sour milk products; tofu; thermally cold drinks like black or green tea, wheat beer, mineral water, thermally cold fruit juices like orange juice; tomatoes, cucumbers, tropical fruits, oranges, lemons, bananas, kiwis, pineapple, watermelon, an excess of spicy and sweet flavors (refined sugar)!

Recommended:

Preparation methods	Neutral and warming
Fish	Warming types of fish such as salmon, trout, tuna, shellfish
Meat	Beef (beef bouillon), chicken (chicken broth), lamb
Fruit	Sweet cherries, plums, peaches, sweet apples, jujubes, apricots, dates, figs, red grapes
Dried fruit	Raisins, figs, prunes, dates, apricots
Vegetables	Warming vegetables like fennel, carrots, sweet potatoes, pumpkin, sautéed onions, cabbage
Beverages	Fennel tea, spice tea with cinnamon, mead, liqueurs, malt beer, licorice tea, red grape juice, corn silk tea
Grains	Millet, oats, sweet rice, rice, buckwheat, amaranth, polenta
Spices	Cayenne pepper, ginger, cinnamon, cardamom, nutmeg, vanilla, star anise, anise, fennel seed, but also spices of the fire phase like coriander, oregano, rosemary, thyme
Nuts and seeds	Pine nuts, pistachios, peanuts, hazelnuts, coconuts, sesame
Sweeteners	Honey, raisins, barley malt, maple syrup, cane sugar

Tip: Generally recommended are the sweet–warm and sweet–hot flavors for strengthening the earth phase; also neutral foods. Regular food intake is important: at least one warm meal a day!

Short-term Fatigue, Feebleness
Spleen Yang Vacuity (Pi Yang Xu)

Symptoms

As in spleen *qi* vacuity, but in addition, cold extremities (constantly cold hands and feet), deeper-lying weakness, chronic fatigue and chills, frequent sensation of cold in the abdomen.

Tongue: Pale, swollen (dental impressions along the edge); slimy moist white fur

Pulse: Deep, slow, faint

Causes

Mostly develops out of chronic spleen *qi* vacuity or from severe weakening of the spleen (pathogenesis as in spleen *qi* vacuity).

Therapy

Strengthen and warm spleen *yang*

激 As in spleen *qi* vacuity with stronger needling technique and Moxa

Avoid:

See p. 210, Spleen *Qi* Vacuity.

Recommended:

See p. 210, Spleen *Qi* Vacuity.

Short-term Fatigue, Feebleness, Blockage
Liver Qi Stagnation (Gan Qi Yu Jie)

Symptoms

Irritability with inner tension, fatigue, flatulence, mental depression, frustration, mood lability, disturbed appetite, globus sensation, PMS, queasiness, nausea, abdominal pain.

Tongue: Blue-black coloration, occasionally rolled up at the edges

Pulse: Tense

Causes

Arises mostly as the result of suppressing emotions like rage, anger, or resentment, which obstruct *qi* circulation.

Therapy

Regulate the flow of liver *qi*
Disperse stagnation

激 • LR-3 • LI-4 • LR-14 • LR-13 • GB-34

Avoid:

All heat-engendering foods!

Recommended:

Only a limited indication exists for Chinese dietetics. Strong flavors or severely *yang*-supplementing foods are able to disperse stagnation. We can often see this in clinic when patients with stagnation have a strong craving for hot spicy foods to compensate. It is important to consume cooling and *yin*-tonifying foods. In addition, the patient should be made aware of the fact that a permanent improvement of his or her complaints requires changes in lifestyle.

Longer-term Fatigue, Exhaustion
Kidney Yang Vacuity (Shen Yang Xu)

Symptoms

Fatigue, feebleness, loss of concentration, chills. Aversion to cold, dizziness, tinnitus, defective hearing, nocturia, edemas, incontinence, morning diarrhea (5 a.m.), loss of libido, impotence; also chronic gastrointestinal disorders.

Tongue: Pale, slack, possibly thin white fur
Pulse: Deep, slow, faint

Causes

In addition to constitutional *yang* vacuity, the causes lie primarily in lifestyle and nutrition. Hence, stress, overwork, lack of sleep, excessive sexual activity, births too close together, and an excess of negative emotions play a large role. An excess of thermally cold foods, *yin* products, irregular food intake, iced drinks, and eating canned food are additional factors. Exposure to cold also contributes.

Therapy

Strengthen and warm kidney *yang* and the *ming men*

激 • KI-7 • GV-4 • CV-4 • CV-6 • BL-23 + Moxa

Strengthen the *ming men*

激 • GV-4 + Moxa

Avoid:

All thermally cool or cold foods, frozen food, raw food, salads, sour milk products, thermally cold fruit and drinks. In addition, refined sugar and alcohol have a strong weakening effect on kidney *qi*.

Recommended:

Thermal nature	Neutral, warm, moderately hot
Flavor	Hot–salty, warm–salty, neutral–salty
Fish	Trout, lobster, salmon, smoked fish
Meat	Game meats (especially venison), pigeon, duck, pork
Vegetables	Fennel, cabbage, leeks, horseradish, root vegetables, onions
Grains	Millet, rice, sweet rice, buckwheat, oats
Nuts and seeds	Chestnuts, black sesame, sunflower seeds, roasted walnuts
Spices	Ginger, garlic, black pepper, cinnamon

Tip: **A good breakfast is important: warm grain porridge, millet, and oats. At least two warm meals a day, use of pungent *yang* spices and *yang* cooking methods (grilling, roasting with alcohol). Master Soup (see p. 33) with warming types of meat, vegetables, and spices!**

■ Longer-term Fatigue, Exhaustion, Burnout

Kidney Yin Vacuity (Shen Yin Xu)

Causes

All factors that cause a kidney *qi* or kidney *yang* vacuity over a longer period of time or with greater intensity eventually end up in kidney *yin* vacuity. Factors that strongly affect the formation of this syndrome are chronic consuming illnesses with states of high fever, excessive use of drugs and alcohol, severe blood loss, extreme stress, and chronic lack of sleep (beware: night shifts, night work).

Symptoms

States of severe exhaustion, burnout syndrome, chronic consuming illnesses, nephritis, spermatorrhea, constitutional weakness, chronic headache, night sweating, frequently in conjunction with the five hot surfaces: hot feet, hot hands, heat and burning behind the sternum. Additionally, we see dry mouth, dry throat, thirst, back and bone pain, tinnitus, defective hearing, dizziness, forgetfulness, impotence, infertility, premature ejaculation.

Tongue: Red, cracked, without fur
Pulse: Vacuous, rapid, stringlike

Therapy

Strengthen kidney *yin*
Conserve and support *yin*
激 • KI-3 • BL-23 • CV-4 • GV-20 • ST-36 • BL-10 • GB-19 • SP-6 • BL-60

Avoid:

Yang-stimulating foods and preparation methods; bitter–hot, bitter–warm, spicy–hot, spicy–warm flavors; foods like coffee, black tea, green tea, red wine, hot spices, salt. In addition, avoid strong mental and physical overwork, lack of sleep, stress, excessive sexual activity.

Recommended:

Thermal nature	Neutral and cooling foods that moisten and produce fluids
Flavor	Salty–neutral, salty–cool, sweet–neutral, sweet–cool
Preparation methods	*Yin*-stimulating
Fish	Oysters, mussels, squid
Fruit	Pears, grapes
Vegetables	Asparagus, cabbage, peas
Grain	Primarily wheat, rice, barley, black soy beans
Nuts and seeds	Black sesame, walnuts, lentils

***Foods for the general strengthening of kidney* qi:**

Fish	Salmon, lobster, tuna, shrimp, smoked fish
Meat	Especially venison and boar, pigeon
Grains	Wheat, millet, oats, black soy beans
Nuts and seeds	Black sesame, walnuts, lentils

Tip: In our culture, we often underestimate the harmful effect of the bitter–warm drug, coffee. Large amounts of coffee consumption in particular dry out the fluids and, over time, damage kidney *yin*. Note: a typical symptom of kidney *yin* vacuity are deep, dark eye rims.

Tip: Strengthening and building kidney *yin* and warming kidney *yang* with appropriate foods tonifies the entire *yin* and *yang* of the organism. Since all diseases with a chronic course ultimately lead to vacuity of kidney *qi*, we often recommend including the kidneys in the treatment concept, similar to the supporting therapy for the center burner.

■ Longer-term Fatigue, Exhaustion, Burnout

Liver Yin Vacuity (Gan Yin Xu)

General

As a syndrome, liver *yin* vacuity rarely appears in isolated symptoms. It is usually combined with the following syndromes: ascendant liver *yang*, life fire flaming upward, and blood vacuity or liver blood vacuity, usually in combination with kidney *yin* vacuity.

Symptoms

Nervousness, fatigue, exhaustion, inner disquietude, dry eyes, dizziness, headache, red face, red cheeks, hot hands and soles of the feet (typical sign of *yin* vacuity), vision disorders, mental depression.

Tongue: Reddish, dry
Pulse: Thin, rapid, stringlike

Therapy

Nurture liver *yin*

激
- LR-3 • GV-20 • GB-20 • GV-16 • LR-8
- SP-6 • furthermore, SI-3 and BL-62
- for women combine with LU-7 and KI-6

Avoid:

Any hot and warm foods, *yang* preparation methods, especially bitter–hot, spicy–hot, sour–hot; all foods that further weaken *yin*, especially strong spices, coffee, high-proof alcohol, red wine, smoking.

Recommended:

Thermal nature	Cool, cold, and neutral foods
Flavor	Sour–refreshing, sour–cool, sour–neutral, sweet–cool, sweet–cold
Preparation methods	*Yin*-strengthening
Vegetables	Tomatoes, cucumbers, spinach, root celery (celeriac), sauerkraut
Beverages	Bread juice
Grains	Wheat, spelt, barley
Dairy products	Sour milk products
Soy products	Tofu

Tip: A balanced diet with neutral and slightly *yin* foods as well as the avoidance of excess *yang* foods, in addition to other changes in lifestyle, can improve these symptoms quite well.

■ Longer-term Fatigue, Exhaustion, Burnout

Liver Blood Vacuity (Gan Xue Xu)

Symptoms

Lusterless face, pronounced paleness, dizziness, unclear vision, dry eyes, night blindness, general feeling of weakness, numbness in the extremities, tremor, cramping, paresthesia, menstrual disorders, weak menstrual period, prolonged with bright red blood, amenorrhea, sleeplessness, loss of concentration, forgetfulness.

Tongue: Pale, small
Pulse: Faint, vacuous

Causes

Malnutrition and insufficient construction of spleen *qi* and liver *yin*, as well as an excess of spicy and *yang*-stimulating foods that weaken the body's *yin*, on occasion also excessively cold foods that reduce spleen *qi*, severe loss of blood, e.g., after surgery or childbirth, all factors that can lead to spleen *qi* or spleen *yang* vacuity as well as kidney *qi* or kidney *yang* vacuity. Excessive activity during the night. Blood is an important *yin* substance that is primarily built by a healthy spleen function, but also by a healthy kidney function. The liver stores and regenerates the blood at night. Disturbing influences on the three viscera, spleen, kidney, and liver, over a longer period of time cause blood vacuity. Because blood is the means by which *qi* is transported, this weakens the entire organism. Problems with the sinews, muscles, and nails result from malnutrition due to blood vacuity. For the *shen*, lastly, the blood serves as resting place, and it can therefore not be anchored securely in patients with liver blood vacuity.

Therapy

Build blood, liver blood

激 • LI-8 • SP-6 • BL-17 • SP-10

Nourish kidney *yin* and liver *yin*

激 • CV-4 • CV-6 • SP-6

Strengthen spleen *qi* and kidneys

激 • SP-2 • SP-3 • BL-20 • BL-21 • ST-36 • KI-3

Psychological

激 • HT-7 • HT-7 • PC-7 • BL-15 • ear *shen men*

Avoid:

Avoid all bitter foods, especially the flavors bitter–hot and bitter–warm, because they dry out the blood. Likewise, the spicy–hot and spicy–warm flavors. In general, patients with blood vacuity should avoid all energetically hot foods. Contraindicated are: coffee, black tea, cocoa, hot spices, such as garlic, ginger, pepper, curry, cinnamon, and so on, energetically hot drinks like high-proof alcohol or yogi tea.

Recommended:

To build spleen qi:	
Flavor	Sweet–neutral, sweet–warm
Fruit	Pears, star fruit, tangerines
Vegetables	Radish, asparagus, water chestnuts, lotus root, dandelion, Chinese (napa) cabbage
Grains	Millet, rice, rye, buckwheat
Spices	Fresh ginger, marjoram, pepper, cardamom
Nuts and seeds	Apricot seeds, almonds, walnuts
To build blood:	
Thermal nature	Warm, neutral
Flavor	Sweet–neutral, sweet–warm
Fish	Squid in its own ink, oysters, mussels
Meat	Especially chicken meat and chicken liver, beef and beef liver, lamb liver, veal liver, chicken soup, beef broth, chicken
Fruit	Sweet–warm, sweet–neutral flavor, red fruits like red grapes and sweet cherries
Vegetables	All thermally neutral and refreshing vegetables, especially red-colored ones like beets and red cabbage
Beverages	Red grape juice, sweet cherry juice, prune juice, red beet juice, red tea (e.g., rose hip, hibiscus), in moderate amounts red wine
Grains	Sweet rice, rice, amaranth

Liver blood vacuity:

Fish	Oysters, prawns, white fish
Meat	Chicken
Grains	Especially wheat and sweet rice
Fruit	Apples
Vegetables	Thermally neutral and refreshing vegetables, especially those associated with the wood phase, which are green in color: spinach, Swiss chard, broccoli, beans; tomatoes; salad: in small amounts mache (corn salad, lamb's lettuce), sprouts
Other	Marjoram, turnip-rooted parsley, egg yolk, water-cress, lotus root, lychees, carrot juice

Longer-term Fatigue, Exhaustion, Burnout

Blood Vacuity—Lack of Blood (Xue Xu)

Symptoms

Blood vacuity is an important pattern in Chinese pathophysiology and is commonly seen in clinical practice. This pattern of disharmony most frequently affects women; men only rarely. From the perspective of Chinese physiology, women have more blood than *qi* and because of menstruation are more closely tied to the reconstruction of blood than men. Blood vacuity is frequently the cause of many gynecological disorders. Men have more *qi* than blood and are more likely to suffer from *qi* problems. The patients are chronically tired and exhausted.

Tongue: Typically a pale, small, dry tongue body
Pulse: Thin, fine, or rough

Therapy

Strengthen the blood, build spleen *qi*, strengthen liver blood

激 • SP-2 • SP-3 • SP-6 • BL-17 • BL-20 • BL-21 • HT-7

Avoid:
See p. 215, Liver Blood Vacuity.

Recommended:
See p. 215, Liver Blood Vacuity.

Cardiovascular Disorders

General Weakness, Lack of Energy, Low Blood Pressure

Brief fatigue, exhaustion	*Spleen qi or spleen yang vacuity*
Lethargy, low blood pressure, dizziness	*Blood vacuity*
Chronic fatigue	*Kidney qi or kidney yang vacuity*

According to TCM:
No direct analogy, often appears in connection with dizziness, headaches, and lethargy. Responds very well to regular and supplementing nutritional therapy, moxibustion, and acupuncture, and possibly herbal therapy.

Therapy

Supplement kidneys, spleen, and stomach
Replenish blood

激 Supplement spleen and stomach:
• ST-36 + Moxa • CV-3 + Moxa
• CV-6 + Moxa • CV-12 + Moxa
Supplement kidneys:
• KI-3 + Moxa • KI-7 + Moxa
• BL-23 + Moxa
Replenish blood:
• ST-36 • CV-4 • SP-6
• LR-8 • BL-17 • BL-20

Avoid:
Coffee, which brings only brief improvement and is especially damaging (drying) to blood (blood vacuity). Thermally cool or cold foods (e.g., raw foods, salads, fruit juices). Excess dairy products, irregular diet, cold meals, or uncooked foods, insufficient use of spices.

Recommended:
Choose foods that supplement spleen, stomach, and kidney and that have a warming and briefly hot effect.

Organ network	Spleen, stomach, kidney
Flavor/thermal nature	Sweet–warm, sweet–hot, salty–warm, salty–hot (not for blood vacuity)
Preparation	Stews simmered for a long time, fried, grilled
Supplement spleen and stomach qi and yang:	
Meat	Duck, lamb, chicken, beef
Fish	Bass, salmon, tuna, eel
Fruit	Cherries, peaches
Vegetables	Fennel, carrots, dates
Grains	Short-grain (glutinous) rice, corn, millet, oats
Spices	Chili, ginger, garlic, pepper, cinnamon, possibly cooking with alcohol
Nuts and seeds	Chestnuts, walnuts
To supplement stomach, spleen, and blood:	
Meat	Chicken, beef
Beverages	Grape juice
Grains	Oats, rice
To supplement kidneys, qi, and yang:	
Meat	Venison, lamb
Fish	Mussels, oysters, sardines
Fruit	Raisins, cherries
Vegetables	Fennel

Grains	Oats, corn
Spices	Honey
Nuts and seeds	Chestnuts, walnuts

Short-term stimulation of heart qi and heart yang:

Beverages	Coffee, cocoa, black tea

Eat regularly, have an ample breakfast, for example oatmeal. Eat more warm, fried, and grilled dishes, such as prawns with garlic and alcohol, and acrid venison and lamb dishes. Increase consumption of meat, simmered soups, or stews with beef or chicken. Increase use of warming spices.

For vegetarians:
Increase use of more supplementing and warming types of grain, for example oats, rice, and corn, with warming acrid spices or vegetables such as leek, ginger, garlic, carrots, and lentils.

Main Symptom: Hypertension (High Blood Pressure)

Hypertension with headache	*Ascendant liver yang (gan yang shang kang)* *Liver fire (gan huo)* *Liver wind (gan feng)*
Hypertension with headache	*Liver yin vacuity and blood vacuity*
Hypertension with tinnitus	*Kidney yin vacuity*
Hypertension with feeling of heaviness	*Phlegm and moisture retention*

According to TCM:
No direct analogy to hypertension. Treatment often in connection with headache or dizziness. Caused by ascending yang, often rooted in liver yin vacuity or kidney yin vacuity. Limited treatment possibilities if hypertension has not manifested for more than one or two years. Recommended treatment: Combination of acupuncture, herbs, and nutritional therapy, combined with conventional allopathic medicine.
Important: *Weight reduction!*

Hypertension with Headache

Ascendant Liver Yang (Gan Yang Shang Kang), Liver Fire (Gan Huo), Liver Wind (Gan Feng)

Symptoms

Hypertension, hypertensive crisis, irritability, anger, insomnia, severe headaches, reddened eyes, tinnitus, reddened face, dry mouth, bitter taste in mouth.

Tongue: Red; white or yellow fur
Pulse: Lateral

Causes

Inappropriate diet (thermally hot foods, alcoholic beverages), often in combination with protracted, heavy emotional burdens, anger, rage, or stress can transform stagnant liver *qi* into ascending liver *yang*, in part also caused by external pathogenic factors such as wind.

Therapy

Downbear ascending *yang*
Calm liver
激 • LR-2 • GB-20 • GB-43 • SI-20 • LR-3 • LI-4

Avoid:
Thermally warm and hot foods, especially acrid spices; alcoholic beverages, bitter–hot foods that damage liver *yin* (such as coffee), acrid foods, especially garlic.

Recommended:
Foods that supplement liver blood and *yin* to drain the ascending *yang* and regulate liver *qi* flow.

Organ network	Liver
Flavor/thermal nature	Sour–neutral, sour–cool, sour–cold, possibly a little sweet–cool and salty–cool
To cool liver heat and drain yang:	
Fruit	Apples, pears, oranges
Vegetables	Wheat, mung beans, spinach
Beverages	Green tea
Dairy products	Milk
To regulate liver qi and downbear qi:	
Fish	Crab, octopus
Fruit	Blueberries, lemons

Vegetables	Dandelion, spinach, celery, tomatoes water chestnuts
Beverages	Chinese chrysanthemum blossom tea, green tea
To supplement liver yin and blood:	
Meat	Duck, pork, chicken
Fruit	Grapes
Vegetables	Spinach, celery, tomatoes
Grains	Black soy beans
Nuts and seeds	Pine nuts, black sesame, sunflower seeds

Green tea, Chinese chrysanthemum blossom tea, freshly cooked wheat porridge, fresh celery juice, tomato juice, apple juice, pear juice. Reduce meat consumption for three weeks or longer.

Hypertension with Headache
Liver Yin Vacuity and Blood Vacuity

Symptoms

Hypertension, dizziness (mild, but persistent), tinnitus, numbness in extremities, heat sensation on palms and soles of feet, insomnia, blurred vision, dry eyes, amenorrhea, scant menstruation, muscle weakness, dry, brittle nails.

Tongue: Reddish; light yellowish fur

Pulse: Fast, thin

Causes

Often appears in people of advanced age in combination with kidney *yin* vacuity, too little sleep at night, overwork, strong emotional burden, inappropriate diet (e.g., excess alcohol, overly acrid foods).

Therapy

Nourish liver *yin*
Drain ascending liver *yang*
激 • LR-3 • BL-18 • LR-8
• KI-3

Avoid:
Thermally hot and drying foods (e.g., coffee, acrid spices, excess salt), excess bitter foods (e.g., coffee, black tea).

Recommended:
Foods that nourish liver *yin* and blood.

Organ network	Liver
Flavor/thermal nature	Sour–neutral, sour–cool, sweet–neutral, sweet–cool
Preparation methods	Boiled, steamed, raw
To clear heat (cooling):	
Vegetables	Dandelion, mung beans, spinach, tomatoes
Beverages	Green tea
To nourish liver yin:	
Meat	Rabbit, pork
Fruit	Mulberries, plums, lemons
Vegetables	Spinach, celery, tomatoes, brown seaweed
Grains	Black soy beans, wheat
Oils and fats	Olive oil
To supplement blood:	
Fruit	Cherries, grapes
Nuts and seeds	Pine nuts

Green tea (too much is drying), freshly ground, cooked wheat porridge, fresh celery juice; meat dishes in moderation, for example beef liver, rabbit liver, pork liver; or, preferably, fish (bass, eel, oysters)

Hypertension with Tinnitus

Kidney Yin Vacuity

Symptoms

Hypertension, sleep disturbances, memory loss, back pain and knee pain, tinnitus, dizziness, impotence, nocturnal ejaculation.

Tongue: Reddish, chapped; little fur
Pulse: Thin, fast

Causes

Too little sleep at night, overwork, sexual excesses, drugs.

Therapy

Supplement kidney *yin*
激 • KI-3 • BL-23 • ST-36 • SP-6 • CV-6 • CV-4 • SI-20

Avoid:

Excess salt; bitter foods, for example coffee and tea; foods with hot thermal nature and acrid flavor, for example garlic, cinnamon, alcohol.

Recommended:

Foods that nourish liver *yin* and essence (*jing*). Possibly also supplement liver *yin*. For heat vacuity symptoms: cool kidney and liver if needed.

Organ network	Liver, kidney
Flavor/thermal nature	Sweet–neutral, sweet–cool, possibly briefly sweet–warm, salty–cool, sour–cool, sour–neutral

To nourish kidney yin:

Meat	Duck, chicken, pork
Fish	Oysters, bass, carp, octopus
Fruit	Cherries, mulberries, raisins, grapes
Grains	Millet, wheat
Dairy products	Butter, cream
Nuts and seeds	Chestnuts, black sesame, walnuts

To nourish liver yin:

Meat	Rabbit, pork
Fruit	Plums, mulberries, lemons
Vegetables	Brown seaweed, spinach, celery, tomatoes
Grains	Black soy beans, wheat
Oils and Fats	Olive oil

Clear heat (cooling):

Fruit	Apples, kiwis
Vegetables	Mung beans, asparagus
Beverages	Green tea, wheat beer

Millet porridge with raisins; freshly ground, cooked wheat porridge, nourishing soup stocks with duck, pork, or chicken. Increase consumption of fish and seafood, for example octopus, oysters, carp, or bass.

Hypertension with Feeling of Heaviness

Retention of Phlegm and Damp

Symptoms

Hypertension, feeling of heaviness in head and extremities; slowed, "dragging" movement; feeling of pressure in chest, dizziness, fatigue, excess weight.

Tongue: Pale; thick white slimy fur
Pulse: Slippery

Causes

Primarily due to inappropriate diet (e.g., excess fatty meat, dairy products, sweets), weakening of spleen, obesity, stress, and overexertion.

Therapy

Dispel moisture and phlegm
Supplement spleen
激 • SP-9 • ST-40 • ST-36 • CV-12 • PC-6 • BL-20 • BL-21 • SP-2

Avoid:

Raw foods, foods with cold thermal nature (fruit, fruit juices, salads), fatty types of meat, too much dairy or citrus fruit, too many sweets (sugar especially promotes the formation of phlegm and damp).

Recommended:

Foods that supplement the spleen, are drying, drain fluids, and transform phlegm.

Organ network	Spleen, stomach
Flavor/thermal nature	Sweet–warm, sweet–neutral, bitter–neutral, bitter–warm, salty–neutral, salty–warm, possibly briefly acrid–neutral, acrid–warm
To transform phlegm and damp:	
Vegetables	Radish
Grains	Barley, soy beans
Spices	Ginger, cardamom, garlic (warm: use sparingly), coriander
To nourish spleen:	
Meat	Beef, lamb
Fruit	Raisins
Vegetables	Beans, fennel, carrots, potatoes
Grains	Oats, rice, corn
Spices	Aniseed, ginger

Transform damp and phlegm:
Porridge of short-grain (glutinous) rice, increase consumption of soy bean products and rice dishes with acrid flavor to transform damp and phlegm: garlic, ginger, coriander, cardamom.

Nourish spleen:
Warm porridge in the morning, for example oats with raisins and cinnamon; corn dishes; stock and stews simmered for a long time with carrots, beef, poultry, acrid spices; fennel tea.

Eye Disorders

Inflammation

According to TCM:
"Fire eye" (red and swollen eyes), often in spring and fall, caused by external wind–heat with repletion conditions in liver and gallbladder (allergy).
Very good results can be achieved by combining acupuncture, nutritional therapy, and herbal therapy.

■ Conjunctivitis

Wind–Heat

Symptoms

Itching and foreign-body sensation in eyes, red swollen eyes, headache, aversion to wind.

Tongue: Reddened sides; thin yellow fur
Pulse: Fast

Causes

External wind–heat and draft during spring or fall that irritate the eyes; wind–heat in the lung pathway, often in combination with heat conditions in liver and gallbladder.

Therapy

Expel external wind–heat
Clear heat
Calm liver
激 • LI-11 • LI-4 • LU-11 • GB-20 • GB-14 • LR-2 • LR-3 • ST-2

Avoid:

Thermally warm and hot foods, acrid spices, alcoholic beverages, grilled foods, and foods fried or seared at high temperatures.

Recommended:

Thermal nature	Cool and cold
Organ network	Liver, gallbladder
Flavor	Bitter, sour, salty, possibly a little sweet
Preparation methods	Raw, boiled, steamed
To expel wind–heat:	
Vegetables	Chinese (napa) cabbage, dandelion, tomatoes
To cool heat:	
Vegetables	Cucumbers, mung beans, spinach, tomatoes, water chestnuts
Beverages	Gentian tea, green tea, wheat beer
Spices	Chinese chrysanthemum blossoms, peppermint

Increase consumption of green tea, mixture of tomato juice and melon juice, Chinese chrysanthemum blossom tea.

Skin Disorders

According to TCM:
General disorder of lung organ network and defense qi, usually both from invasion of pathogenic factors such as wind, heat, damp, dryness. Other contributing factors: Emotions and inappropriate diet.

Neurodermatitis

Acute flare-up	*Wind–heat, heat in blood*
Chronic condition	*Blood vacuity and dryness*

According to TCM:

Combination of external pathogenic factors, such as wind, heat, dryness, emotional imbalance, and inappropriate diet.
Good therapeutic results can be achieved with dietary measures in combination with acupuncture and herbs.

■ Acute Flare-Up
Wind–Heat, Heat in Blood

Symptoms
Red, itching skin with flat pustules, partly oozing; crust formation, scaling, restlessness, irritability, hyperactivity.
Tongue: Pale, in part with red, raised dots; possibly thin, yellow fur
Pulse: Rapid

Causes
External wind–heat penetrating skin, heat stagnation, enduring emotional strain and inappropriate diet causing heat in blood.

Therapy

Expel wind–heat
Dispel heat in blood
激 • LI-11 • SP-10 • SP-6
• GV-14 • BL-40 • LR-2 • GB-43

Avoid:
Thermally warm and hot foods, acrid spices.

Recommended:

Thermal nature	Cool and cold
Organ network	Liver, lung
Flavor	Sour, a little sweet, a little bitter
To dispel wind–heat:	
Vegetables	Chinese (napa) cabbage, carrots, dandelion, radish, tomatoes
To cool blood:	
Vegetables	Brown seaweed, mung beans, tomatoes, spinach, celery
Beverages	Green tea, wheat beer
Grains	Wheat
To moisten dryness:	
Fruit	Bananas, pears, kiwis, watermelons
Grains	Soy beans, wheat
Spices	Honey
Nuts and seeds	Peanuts, pine nuts

Dairy products	Butter, yogurt, kefir, cream
Soy products	Soy milk, tofu

Wind–heat and heat in blood:
Increase consumption of green tea; dandelion decoction, Belgian endive hearts salad.

Moisten dry skin:
Pear juice, baked bananas, increase consumption of soy milk products.

■ Chronic Conditions

Blood Vacuity and Dryness

Symptoms

Dry, dull skin with heavy scaling, possibly occasional itching (due to internal liver wind), pale lips, dizziness, forgetfulness, depression, amenorrhea, chronic symptoms.

Tongue: Pale, pink, small
Pulse: Thin, deep

Causes

Vacuity of body fluids, for example from enduring heat, inappropriate diet, or wind–dryness, weakens the blood and leads to blood vacuity.

Therapy

Supplement blood
Moisten dryness
Calm liver wind
激 • LR-3 • SP-6 • SP-10 • ST-36 • KI-6 • GV-14

Avoid:
Thermally hot foods; highly drying foods with bitter taste, for example coffee, black tea, acrid spices, too much salt.

Recommended:

Thermal nature	Blood heat: cool, cold Blood vacuity: neutral, cool, a little warm
Organ network	Liver, lung
Flavor	Sweet, a little sour
Preparation	Boiled, steamed, baked
To supplement blood:	
Meat	Duck, chicken, liver, beef
Fish	Bass, octopus
Fruit	Cherries, plums, grapes
Nuts and seeds	Pine nuts, black sesame
Other	Chicken eggs
To cool blood heat:	
Fish	Oysters
Vegetables	(Brown seaweed), dandelion, spinach, celery, tomatoes
To nourish yin:	
Fish	Eel
Vegetables	Carrots, potatoes
Grains	Wheat, spelt
Spices	Honey
Dairy products	Butter, cow's milk, cow's milk cheese

Acne

According to TCM:
"Damp-heat which slumbers inside the skin." Consistent dietary measures, in combination with acupuncture and herbal therapy, can achieve very good and lasting results.

Common Acne

Damp–Heat, Possibly Liver Qi Vacuity Combined with Binding Depression of Liver Qi (Gan Qi Yu Jie)

Symptoms
Reddened to yellowish pustules on skin; impure, oily skin, inflammation, fatigue, exhaustion (with spleen *qi* vacuity), irritability, sleep disturbances (with heat, liver *qi* stagnation).
Tongue: Swollen; thick yellow fur
Pulse: Weak

Causes
Primarily inappropriate diet (e.g., excess of sweet, fatty, and thermally hot foods), emotional imbalance causing internal heat and intensified by inappropriate diet; spleen *qi* vacuity causes dampness.

Therapy

Dispel heat and dampness
Supplement spleen
激 • LI-11 • LI-4 • GB-20 • LR-3
• SP-10 • GV-10 • SP-6 • LU-5

Avoid:
Thermally hot and fatty foods (junk food), especially acrid spices (garlic, ginger, pepper), grilled and smoked meat; sweets; meat consumption; with weak spleen, consumption of dairy products.

Recommended:
Select foods that cool heat and remove dampness, calm and cool the liver, and supplement the spleen without creating heat and dampness.

Thermal nature/flavor	Sour–neutral, sour–cool, bitter–neutral, bitter–cool, possibly briefly bitter–cold and sour–cold, sweet–neutral
Organ network	Liver, gallbladder, spleen
To expel dampness and heat:	
Fruit	Pears, tangerines
Vegetables	Mung beans, asparagus
Beverages	Corn silk tea, green tea, black tea
To cool heat:	
Vegetables	Belgian endive hearts, dandelion, mung beans
Beverages	Gentian tea
Grains	Wheat
Soy products	Tofu
For liver stagnation, to move and cool blood:	
Vegetables	Radish, spinach, celery, tomatoes
Other	Vinegar
To supplement spleen:	
Meat	Poultry, beef
Fruit	Apples
Vegetables	Eggplant, cucumbers, carrots, fennel
Grains	Spelt, barley, millet, rice, wheat
Nuts and seeds	Almonds, black sesame
Soy products	Tofu

Tea cure:
For three to six weeks, drink 1 L (four cups) of corn silk tea daily. Increase consumption of green or black tea, millet porridge, and fresh vegetables, for example spinach, salads with mung bean sprouts, bamboo sprouts, tomatoes; give preference to spelt products.

Urogenital Disorders

Main Symptom: Cystitis (Urinary Tract Infections/Inflammation)

Nonbacterial cystitis	*Damp–cold in bladder*
Bacterial cystitis	*Damp–heat in bladder*

According to TCM:
Damp–cold or damp–heat often accumulate from external pathogenic sources, primarily cold in the lower burner (bladder). Good therapeutic results for recurrent cystitis can be achieved with acupuncture and nutritional therapy.

■ Nonbacterial Cystitis
Damp–Cold in Bladder

Symptoms
Frequent desire to urinate with light, cloudy urine, sometimes difficult micturition, feeling of heaviness in hypogastrium (lower abdomen).
Tongue: White, sticky fur at the root of the tongue
Pulse: Slippery

Causes
Overall lowered resistance (*qi* and *yang* vacuity, in part of the kidneys), often caused by external pathogenic cold, possibly following emotional strain, for example fear; excessive sexual activity weakens kidney *yang*.

Therapy

Remove dampness
Dispel cold
Supplement bladder and kidneys
激 • SP-9 • SP-6 • CV-3 • CV-9 • DV4 • BL-23 • KI-7

Avoid:
Foods with cool and cold thermal nature, dairy products, excess meat.

Recommended:
Foods that remove dampness, supplement the lower burner, supplement kidney *yang*, and nourish the spleen.

Organ network	Kidney, bladder, spleen
Flavor/thermal nature	Bitter–neutral, bitter–warm, sweet–neutral, sweet–warm
Preparation methods	Boiled, fried
To expel dampness:	
Fish	Carp, bass
Vegetables	Adzuki beans
Grains	Corn
Spices	Ginger, garlic
To supplement spleen:	See "Spleen/pancreas Network," page 67
To nourish kidney yang:	
Fish	Prawns, eel
Meat	Venison, lamb, poultry
Fruit	Cherries, raspberries
Vegetables	Fennel
Beverages	Corn silk tea
Grains	Millet, corn, oats
Spices	Cloves, cinnamon, rosemary, fennel
Nuts and seeds	Chestnuts, walnuts, black sesame

Start by removing fluids, for example with corn silk tea, adzuki beans, more soy products; then supplement spleen and kidneys with warming dishes such as millet porridge with raisins and cinnamon, acridly spiced rice dishes, acridly spiced meat dishes, fennel tea.

Bacterial Cystitis

Damp–Heat in Bladder

Symptoms

Frequent desire to urinate with burning sensation during urination; dark yellow, cloudy urine; hematuria (blood in urine), fever, thirst.
Tongue: Red; thick, yellow, and sticky fur
Pulse: Fast, sliding

Causes

Exposure to external damp–heat or damp–cold that turns into heat, heavy emotional burden, weakened resistance.

Therapy

Disperse heat
Expel dampness
Open waterways of the lower burner

激 • CV-4 • SP-9 • SP-6
• BL-39 • BL-66

In combination with conventional, allopathic medicine!

Avoid:

Foods with warm and hot thermal nature (acrid spices, alcoholic beverages), foods that produce dampness and heat (excess sweets, fatty, and thermally hot foods like chips, French fries, coke, junk food).

Recommended:

Foods that cool heat and expel dampness; if needed, nourish spleen and supplement kidney *qi*.

Organ network	Kidney, bladder, spleen
Flavor/thermal nature	Salty–neutral, salty–cool, bitter–neutral, bitter–cool, possibly briefly bitter–cold, sweet–neutral, sweet–cool
To expel damp–heat:	
Vegetables	Adzuki beans, cucumbers, mung bean sprouts, radish, tomatoes, celery
Beverages	Dandelion tea, corn silk tea
Grains	Amaranth, barley
Nuts and seeds	Job's tears
Soy products	Soy milk
To supplement spleen:	
	Use sweet–warm sparingly, better: sweet–neutral (otherwise dampness recurs)
To supplement kidney qi:	
Fruit	Cherries, raspberries
Vegetables	Fennel
Grains	Oats, corn, millet
Spices	Cinnamon, honey, rosemary
Nuts and seeds	Chestnuts, pistachios, walnuts
To cool heat:	
Vegetables	Bamboo sprouts, mung beans
Beverages	Green tea

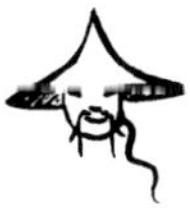

Corn silk tea, dandelion tea, fresh radish juice, or celery juice

Incontinence, Enuresis (Bedwetting), Frequent Micturition (Urination)

Kidney Qi Vacuity, Kidney Yang Vacuity

According to TCM:
Kidney yang vacuity or unstable kidney qi due to weak constitution, advanced age, or excessive sexual activity. In children, "fear," in addition to constitution, is often an initial factor that weakens the kidneys. Good therapeutic results can be achieved by combining nutrition, acupuncture, and herbs.

Symptoms

Urinary stuttering, incontinence, nocturnal incontinence in children, pale urine, nycturia, general weakness, exhaustion, pain in back and knees, dizziness, sexual disorders, psychovegetative (psychosomatic) disorders, cold sensation with *yang* vacuity.

Tongue: Pale, damp
Pulse: Weak, deep

Causes

Weak constitution, advanced age, excessive sexual activity; heavy emotional burden, especially shock and fear, which can traumatize or permanently weaken the kidneys.

Therapy

Supplement and warm kidneys
激
- LI-7 • LI-3 • BL-23 + Moxa
- GV-4 + Moxa • CV-6 + Moxa
- HT-7 • GV-20

Avoid:

Foods with cool and cold thermal nature (raw foods, fruit juices, dairy products).

Recommended:

Foods that supplement kidney *qi* and kidney *yang*.

Organ network	Kidney
Flavor/thermal nature	Sweet–warm, sweet–neutral, possibly sweet–hot (briefly)
Preparation methods	Boiled, fried, grilled
Meat	Venison, poultry, lamb
Fruit	Raspberries, raisins, cherries
Vegetables	Fennel, leeks
Grains	Oats, corn, millet
Spices	Star anise, cinnamon, rosemary
Nuts and seeds	Chestnuts, walnuts, black sesame

Prawns sautéed in alcohol with acrid spices and Chinese leek (garlic chives); fried walnuts with leeks.

Fresh oatmeal with raisins and cinnamon; three to four walnuts daily; acrid meat dishes, for example: venison, lamb, poultry with acrid spices; broth and stews with warming types of meat and acrid spices; fennel tea.

Impotence, Weak Libido

Kidney Yang Vacuity

According to TCM:
Kidney yang vacuity extinguishes kidney fire: ming men ("life gate fire"). TCM believes that the essence (jing) should be conserved and treated with care. Conservation of the seminal fluid (jing) is viewed as health-preserving and life-prolonging. Unnecessary loss of semen and sexual dissipation weaken kidney yang and kidney yin.

Symptoms

Erectile dysfunction (no erection, or erections that last only a few seconds), spermatorrhea, frequent micturition, general exhaustion, back and knee pain, tinnitus, dizziness, blurred vision; dull, pale complexion.

Tongue: Pale; white fur, damp
Pulse: Deep, weak

Causes

Constitutional weakness, overwork, dissipative sex life, emotional stress and fear, inappropriate diet, foods with overly cold and cool thermal nature.

Therapy

Supplement and warm kidney *yang*
Support essence (*jing*)

激
- GV-4 + Moxa • KI-3 • KI-7 + Moxa
- BL-23 + Moxa • CV-4 + Moxa
- ST-36 • GV-20

Avoid:
Raw and thermally cool and cold foods (fruit, salads, raw foods), excess dairy products, sugar, excess coffee, alcoholic beverages, excess acrid spices (prolonged use weakens kidney *yang* and kidney *yin*).

Recommended:
Foods that nourish and warm kidney *qi* and kidney *yang*.

Organ network	Kidney
Flavor/thermal nature	Sweet–warm, sweet–hot, sweet–neutral, acrid–warm, acrid–hot (only briefly)
Preparation methods	Boiled, grilled, fried
Meat	Venison, poultry, lamb, goat, duck
Fish	Eel, shrimp, oysters, mussels
Fruit	Raisins, cherries, raspberries
Vegetables	Fennel, leeks
Grains	Oats, corn
Spices	Rosemary, star anise, cinnamon, garlic, ginger
Nuts and seeds	Chestnuts, pistachios, black sesame, walnuts, lentils

Shrimp fried in alcohol with acrid spices, such as garlic;

Spiced fried or grilled venison, lamb, or poultry;

Simmered stews with supplementing types of meat (Master Soup);

Increased use of acrid spices, for example garlic, cinnamon, chili, and ginger; during winter, roasted chestnuts and roasted walnuts;

Freshly cooked oat porridge with cinnamon and raisins.

Gynecological Disorders

Morning Sickness During Pregnancy

According to TCM:
Vacuity or disharmony of center burner. Very good results are often achieved with dietary measures and acupuncture (PC-6), in severe cases in combination with herbs.

During pregnancy, acupuncture and herbs should only be administered by practitioners with a very good knowledge of these therapies, since some acupuncture points are contraindicated during pregnancy (they increase labor pain, can increase pathological disease progression, and can lead to premature birth). With recurrent vomiting, ensure sufficient intake of fluids, possibly intravenous hydration with fluids by allopathic physician.

■ Morning Sickness during Pregnancy

Spleen and Stomach Qi Vacuity
Stomach and Spleen Yang Vacuity

Symptoms

Vomiting of watery fluids, in part with undigested food particles after meals, loss of appetite, fatigue, heart palpitations.

Tongue: Pale, damp; white fur
Pulse: Slow, slippery

Causes

Vacuity and disharmony of center burner with upbearing stomach *qi*, in part caused by inappropriate diet (excess foods with cold thermal nature), overburden.

Therapy

Supplement spleen and stomach
Downbear counterflow *qi*

激 Only with good knowledge of acupuncture:
- PC-6 (most important point)
- ST-36 • CV-12 • GV-20
- SP-4 • CV-13

Avoid:
Raw and thermally cold and cool foods (salads, fruit, fruit juices), excess dairy, excess of acrid spices.

Recommended:
Foods that supplement spleen and stomach and that downbear *qi*.

Organ network	Spleen, stomach
Flavor/thermal nature	Sweet–warm, sweet–neutral
Preparation methods	Steamed, boiled
Fruit	Dates, raisins
Vegetables	Fennel, carrots, sweet Hpotatoes
Grains	Millet, rice
Spices	Freshly grated ginger, malt

Tip: **A pinch of freshly grated ginger daily in the morning, for one to two weeks!**
Or simmer a thumb-sized piece of fresh ginger in 0.5 L (two cups) of water for 20 minutes; drink while warm.

Rice or millet dishes, possibly with mildly acrid spices, fennel tea, carrot stew, stock from beef and carrots, chicken soup, millet porridge.

Foods that should be avoided during pregnancy, according to TCM:

Acrid–hot foods (lead to heat and commotion in the blood and disturb the fetus). Chili, garlic, cinnamon, lamb, coffee (dries and heats up the blood). Excess black and green tea or red wine (dries the blood). Crab/crayfish (cause too much heat in blood) and citrus fruit (cooling/cold).

Liver Qi Invading the Stomach (Gan Qi Fan Wei)

Symptoms

Vomiting of bitter, sour liquid; sour belching, bitter taste in mouth, strong thirst, tenseness in thorax and hypochondrium region, headaches, dizziness, irritability.

Tongue: Pale, reddened sides; thin, yellow or white fur

Pulse: Slippery

Causes

Stagnation of heat in liver from emotional strain, inappropriate diet (overly acrid and hot foods) lead to repletion heat in the liver and attack the stomach.

Therapy

Calm liver
Supplement and harmonize stomach
Downbear counterflow *qi*

激 Only with a good knowledge of acupuncture:

• PC-6 • ST-36 • CV-12 • LR-3

May induce/promote labor; only with clear indication.

Recommended:

Foods that cool liver heat and calm the liver, harmonize and nourish spleen and stomach *qi*.

Organ network	Liver, spleen, stomach
Flavor/thermal nature	Cool liver heat: sour–cool, sweet–cool
	Harmonize stomach and spleen: sweet–cool, sweet–neutral
Preparation method	Boiled, steamed
To cool liver heat:	
Fruit	Apples, strawberries
Vegetables	Eggplant, mung beans
Grains	Pearl barley, wheat
Beverages	Black tea, green tea
To downbear ascending liver qi:	
Fish	Oysters
Vegetables	Spinach, celery, tomatoes
Beverages	Green tea
To harmonize and supplement stomach and spleen:	
Vegetables	Carrots, sweet potatoes
Grains	Corn, rice, millet
Spices	Honey
Dairy products	Cow's milk
Nuts and seeds	Almonds
For upbearing stomach qi and stomach heat:	
Fruit	Bananas, kiwis, watermelons
Vegetables	Bamboo sprouts, dandelion, water chestnuts
Beverages	Green tea

6 Chinese Dietetics At a Glance

Foods Classified by Phase/Organ Network

土 Phase: Earth
Organ Network: Spleen/Pancreas, Stomach

Food	Thermal Nature	Flavor	Effect
Vegetables			
Beet	Neutral	Sweet, slightly bitter	Balances spleen and stomach *qi*
Cabbage, green	Neutral to warming	Acrid, sweet	Balances stomach, spleen
Cabbage, red	Neutral to warming	Acrid, sweet	Balances spleen, stomach, blood
Carrot	Neutral	Sweet	Supplements center burner
Celery root (celeriac)	Cooling	Sweet, slightly bitter	Liver, cools stomach heat
Mushroom, button, crimini, portobella	Cooling	Sweet	Cools blood and heat
Chili (or chile) pepper, capsicum	Warming	Sweet, slightly acrid, bitter	Moves blood and *qi*
Chinese (napa) cabbage	Neutral to cool-ing	Sweet	Cools heat, diuretic
Cucumber	Cold	Sweet, slightly bitter	Cools heat, diuretic
Eggplant	Cooling	Bitter, slightly sweet	Cools liver heat
Fennel	Warming	Sweet, acrid	Balances *qi*, harmonizes center burner
Lettuce	Cooling to cold	Sweet, slightly bitter	Cools heat
Onion	Warming	Acrid, sweet	Moves *qi*
Parsnip	Neutral to warming	Sweet, bitter, acrid	Balances stomach, intestine, lung
Potato	Neutral	Sweet	Strengthens spleen and stomach *qi*
Pumpkin	Neutral to warming	Sweet	Supplements center burner, strengthens *qi*
Salsify	Cooling	Sweet, slightly bitter	Balances blood and cools
Sweet potato	Neutral to warming	Sweet	Supplements center burner and balances *qi* and blood
Tomato	Cooling to cold	Sweet, sour	Supports liver *yin*
Zucchini	Cooling	Sweet, bitter	Cools stomach heat and liver heat

Food	Thermal Nature	Flavor	Effect
Legumes			
Black bean	Neutral	Sweet	Supplements spleen, kidneys
Chickpea (garbanzo bean)	Neutral	Sweet	Supplements *qi*, spleen, and kidneys
Fava (broad) bean	Neutral	Sweet	Supplements spleen, drains dampness
Green bean (snap bean)	Neutral	Sweet	Supplements blood and *qi*
Lentil, green	Neutral	Sweet	Supplements *qi* and blood
Lentil, red	Neutral to warming	Sweet	Supplements kidney and heart *qi*
Peanut	Neutral	Sweet	Moistens lungs
Snap pea	Neutral to slightly cool	Sweet	Supplements spleen
Snow pea	Neutral	Sweet	Supplements *qi* and blood
Soybean, black	Neutral	Sweet	Supplements spleen, kidneys
Soybean, green	Neutral to cool	Sweet	Cools heat
Soybean sprout	Neutral	Sweet	Expels damp–heat
Tofu	Neutral to cool	Sweet	Cools heat
White bean	Neutral	Sweet	Supplements spleen
Pea, yellow (yellow split pea, dal)	Neutral	Sweet	Supplements spleen
Fruit			
Grape	Neutral to warming	Sweet	Supplements blood and *qi*
Apricot	Neutral to warming	Sweet, sour	Supplements body fluids
Banana	Cold	Sweet	Moistens large intestine
Currant	Cooling	Sweet, sour	Astringent, forms body fluids and blood
Cherry	Warming	Sweet	Supplements body fluids
Cranberry	Cooling to neutral	Sweet, sour	Increases appetite
Currant	Cooling	Sweet, sour	Astringent, forms body fluids and blood
Date	Neutral	Sweet	Supplements blood and body fluids
Elderberry	Cool to neutral	Bitter, sweet	Balances intestine
Fig (fresh)	Neutral to warming	Sweet	Strengthens center burner, moistens
Melon	Cooling	Sweet	Cools heat
Orange	Cooling to cold	Sweet, sour	Supplements body fluids

Food	Thermal Nature	Flavor	Effect
Peach	Neutral to warming	Sweet, sour	Supplements body fluids
Pear	Neutral to cooling	Sweet, slightly sour	Cools stomach heat, moistens
Pineapple	Cooling to neutral	Sweet, sour	Activates digestion
Quince	Neutral to cooling	Slightly bitter	Strengthens intestine
Tangerine	Cooling	Sweet, sour	Cools heat, supplements body fluids
Watermelon	Cold	Sweet	Cools heat
Grains			
Barley	Cooling	Sweet, slightly salty	Drains dampness, cools heat
Buckwheat	Cooling	Sweet, slightly bitter	Strengthens spleen
Corn (maize)	Neutral to warming	Sweet	Supplements *qi* and blood
Millet	Neutral to warming	Sweet, slightly bitter	Supplements *qi* and cools heat
Oats	Neutral to warming	Sweet, slightly bitter	Supplements blood and *qi*
Rice	Neutral to warming	Sweet	Supplements *qi*, strengthens center burner
Rye	Neutral to warming	Sweet, slightly bitter	Supplements and strengthens *qi*
Spelt	Neutral to warming	Sweet	Supplements spleen *qi*
Wheat	Cooling	Sweet	Supplements *qi*, blood, and *yin*
Oils, Fats			
Butter	Neutral to cool	Sweet, fatty	Supplements blood and *qi*, moistens
Lard (pork)	Neutral to cooling	Sweet, fatty	Moistens
Margarine	Neutral	Sweet, fatty	Moistens
Olive oil	Cooling	Sweet, fatty	Moistens
Peanut butter	Neutral	Sweet, fatty	Moistens
Peanut oil	Neutral	Sweet, fatty	Moistens
Soy oil	Neutral to warming	Sweet, fatty	Moistens, laxative
Sesame oil	Neutral to cooling	Sweet, fatty	Moistens skin and intestine
Sunflower oil	Neutral to cooling	Sweet, fatty	Moistens, enriches *yin*

Food	Thermal Nature	Flavor	Effect
Dairy Products			
Butter	Neutral to cool	Sweet, fatty	Supplements blood and *qi*, moistens
Buttermilk	Cooling	Sweet	Moistens, cools heat
Cheese, cow's milk	Neutral	Acrid, salty	Moistens
Cheese, goat's milk	Warming	Acrid, salty	Warms center burner
Cheese, sheep's milk	Warming	Acrid, salty, sweet	Warms center burner
Cream	Neutral	Sweet, fatty	Supplements *qi* and blood, moistens
Cottage cheese	Cooling to cold	Sweet, slightly sour	Moistens
Cream cheese	Cooling	Sweet	Moistens, cools heat
Milk, cow's	Neutral to cooling	Sweet	Moistens, cools
Milk, goat's and sheep's	Neutral to warming	Sweet	Moistens, warms
Sour cream	Neutral to cool	Sour, sweet	Enriches *yin*
Yogurt	Cooling to cold	Sweet, sour	Enriches *yin*, cools intestine
Nuts, Seeds			
Coconut	Cooling	Sweet	Expels heat
Peanut	Neutral to warming	Sweet, fatty	Moistens lung
Peanut butter	Neutral	Sweet, fatty	Moistens
Pistachio	Neutral	Sweet, slightly bitter	Moistens skin and lung
Sesame, black	Neutral	Sweet, fatty	Strengthens liver and kidneys
Sesame, white	Cooling	Sweet, fatty	Supplements blood and body fluids
Meat, Poultry, Eggs			
Beef	Neutral	Sweet	Supplements *qi* and blood
Chicken	Warming	Sweet	Supplements *qi* and blood
Duck	Neutral to cooling	Sweet, slightly salty	Supplements *qi*, blood and *yin*
Egg, chicken	Neutral	Sweet	Supplements blood and *yin*
Goat	Warming	Sweet	Supplements spleen and liver *yang*
Goose	Neutral	Sweet	Supplements spleen *qi*
Hare, wild/rabbit	Neutral to cooling	Sweet	Supplements spleen and *qi*
Pork	Cooling	Sweet, fatty	Supplements blood and *yin*
Veal	Neutral	Sweet	Supplements spleen *qi*

Food	Thermal Nature	Flavor	Effect
Fish			
Bass	Neutral	Sweet, slightly salty	Supplements *qi* and blood
Crab (sweet water)	Cold	Sweet	Enriches *yin*
Eel	Warming	Sweet, fatty	Supplements *qi* and blood
Salmon	Warming	Sweet, slightly salty, fatty	Supplements *qi* and blood
Trout	Neutral to warming	Sweet	Supplements center burner
Spices			
Aniseed	Warming	Acrid, sweet	Stimulates digestion
Caraway	Warming	Acrid, sweet	Stimulates digestion
Chili pepper	Hot	Acrid	Expels cold
Curry	Warming to hot	Acrid, bitter	Stimulates digestion
Fennel seed	Warming	Acrid, sweet	Stimulates digestion
Honey	Neutral	Sweet	Supplements *qi* and blood
Paprika	Mildly warming	Bitter, slightly sweet	Stimulates digestion
Saffron	Neutral to cooling	Sweet, bitter, acrid	Balances liver, spleen
Herbs			
Chamomile	Neutral to cooling	Slightly bitter, sweet	Harmonizes digestion
Corn silk	Cooling	Slightly sweet	Astringent, cools damp–heat
Licorice	Neutral	Very sweet, slightly bitter	Stimulates digestion, supplements center burner
Onion	Warming	Acrid, sweet	Loosens phlegm
Beverages, Alcoholic Beverages			
Beer	Cooling to cold	Bitter, sweet	Cools liver heat
Liqueur	Hot	Acrid, bitter–sweet	Dispels internal cold

金 Phase: Metal
Organ Network: Lung–Large Intestine

Food	Thermal Nature	Flavor	Effect
Vegetables			
Asparagus	Cooling	Sweet, bitter	Supplements kidney *yin* and lungs, diuretic
Cauliflower	Neutral to cool	Sweet, slightly bitter	Cools stomach heat and lungs
Chili pepper	Warming	Sweet, slightly acrid, bitter	Moves *qi* and blood
Fennel	Warming	Sweet, acrid	Balances *qi*, harmonizes center burner
Garden cress	Cooling	Acrid	Balances *qi* and blood
Garlic	Warming to hot	Acrid	Moves *qi*, loosens phlegm
Green onion	Warming	Acrid	Moves *qi*, expels cold
Kohlrabi	Neutral	Acrid, sweet	Supplements liver, gallbladder and kidneys
Leek	Warming	Acrid, sweet	Moves *qi*, warms center burner
Onion	Warming	Acrid, sweet	Moves *qi*
Radish, icicle, daikon (raw)	Neutral to cool	Acrid to mildly acrid (daikon)	Loosens phlegm in lungs and stomach
Radish, small, round	Cooling	Acrid	Loosens blood stagnation, blood heat
Arugula (rocket, rucola) lettuce	Neutral to cooling	Acrid, bitter	Stimulates appetite
Legumes			
Bean, black	Neutral	Sweet	Supplements kidneys and spleen
Oils			
Peanut oil	Neutral	Sweet, fatty	Moistens
Peanut butter	Neutral	Sweet, fatty	Moistens
Nuts, Seeds			
Peanut	Neutral to warming	Sweet, fatty	Moistens lung
Pistachio	Neutral	Sweet, slightly bitter	Moistens skin and lung
Meat, Poultry			
Duck	Neutral to cooling	Sweet, slightly salty	Supplements *qi*, blood, and *yin*

Food	Thermal Nature	Flavor	Effect
Spices			
Caraway seed	Warming	Acrid, sweet	Stimulates digestion
Cardamom	Warming	Acrid, slightly bitter	Stimulates digestion
Cayenne pepper	Hot	Very acrid	Expels cold
Cinnamon bark	Warming to hot	Acrid	Astringent, expels cold
Cinnamon twig	Warming	Acrid, bitter	Stimulates digestive organs
Clove	Warming	Bitter, slightly sweet	Expels damp cold
Coriander	Neutral to cooling	Bitter, acrid	Stimulates digestion
Ginger	Warming to hot	Acrid, slightly sweet	Loosens phlegm
Nutmeg	Warming	Acrid	Astringent, expels damp–heat
Pepper (season-ing), black (ripe)	Warming to hot	Very acrid	Enriches *yang*, expels cold
Pepper (seasoning), green (unripe)	Warming	Acrid	Enriches *yang*, moves *qi*
Pepper (seasoning), white (fully ripe)	Warming to hot	Very acrid	Enriches *yang*, expels cold
Turmeric (curcuma)	Warming	Bitter, acrid	Dries phlegm–cold
Herbs			
Basil	Warming	Acrid, bitter, slightly sweet	Stimulates digestion, loosens phlegm
Garden cress	Cooling	Acrid, slightly bitter	Stimulates digestion, strengthens immune system
Fennel seeds	Warming	Slightly acrid, sweet	Stimulates digestion
Garlic	Warming to hot	Acrid, slightly salty	Dispels phlegm–cold
Horseradish	Warming, heating	Very acrid	Enriches *yang*
Onion	Warming	Acrid, sweet	Loosens phlegm
Sage	Warming	Bitter, acrid	Mildly expels phlegm–cold
Savory	Warming	Acrid, bitter, slightly sweet	Stimulates digestion, loosens phlegm
Thyme	Warming	Bitter, acrid	Dries, moves *qi*, loosens phlegm
Watercress	Warming	Acrid, slightly bitter	Stimulates digestion

Food	Thermal Nature	Flavor	Effect
Alcoholic Beverages			
Liqueur, spirits	Hot	Acrid, bitter, sweet	Dispel internal cold

水 Phase: Water
Organ Network: Kidney–Bladder

Food	Thermal Nature	Flavor	Effect
Vegetables			
Asparagus	Cooling	Sweet, bitter	Supplements lung and kidney *yin*, diuretic
Fruit			
Raspberry	Cooling	Sweet, sour	Mild laxative, diuretic
Strawberry	Cooling	Sweet, sour	Forms body fluids and blood
Grains			
Barley	Cooling	Sweet, slightly salty	Cools heat
Corn (maize)	Neutral to warming	Sweet	Supplements *qi* and blood
Millet	Neutral	Sweet, slightly bitter	Supplements *qi*
Wheat	Cooling	Sweet	Supplements *qi*, blood, and *yin*
Oils			
Walnut oil	Warming	Sweet, fatty	Supplements kidney *yang*
Nuts, Seeds			
Sesame, black	Neutral	Sweet, fatty	Strengthens liver and kidneys
Chestnuts	Warming	Sweet	Strengthens spleen and kidneys
Sunflower seeds	Neutral	Sweet, fatty	Nourishes *yin*, moistening
Walnuts	Warming	Sweet, bitter, fatty	Strengthens lungs and kidneys
Meat			
Goat	Warming	Sweet	Supplements spleen and kidney *yang*
Lamb	Warming to hot	Sweet, slightly bitter	Supplements kidney–spleen *yang*
Pheasant	Warming	Sweet, slightly sour	Supplements center burner
Pork	Cooling	Sweet, fatty	Supplements blood and *yin*
Venison, red deer, blacktailed deer	Warming	Sweet	Supplements *qi*, blood, and *yang*
Venison, reindeer, moose, elk, roe deer	Neutral to warming	Sweet	Supplements *qi* and blood
Wild boar (pig)	Neutral to warming	Sweet	Supplements *qi* and *yang*

Food	Thermal Nature	Flavor	Effect
Fish			
Bass	Neutral	Sweet, slightly salty	Supplements *qi* and blood
Caviar	Cold	Salty	Supplements kidney *yin*
Crab (sweet water)	Cold	Sweet, slightly salty	Enriches *yin*
Crayfish	Cold	Sweet	Enriches *yin*
Eel	Warming	Sweet, fatty	Supplements *qi* and blood
Lobster	Neutral to warming	Sweet, slightly salty	Supplements kidney *qi* and kidney *yang*
Mussel	Warming	Salty	Supplements liver *yang* and kidney *qi* and *yang*
Octopus (squid)	Neutral to cooling	Sweet, salty	Supplements *qi*, blood, and *yin*
Oyster	Neutral to cooling	Sweet, salty	Supplements liver, kidneys, blood, and *yin*
Prawn	Warming	Sweet, slightly salty	Supplements kidney *qi* and kidney *yang*
Salmon	Warming	Sweet, slightly salty, fatty	Supplements *qi* and blood
Sardine	Neutral	Sweet, slightly salty	Supplements *qi* and blood
Sea snail (conch)	Neutral	Sweet, salty	Supplements liver *yin* and kidney *yin*
Trout	Neutral to warming	Sweet	Supplements center burner
Tuna	Neutral to warming	Sweet, slightly salty	Supplements *qi* and blood
Spices			
Miso	Neutral to cooling	Salty, slightly sour	Harmonizes digestion
Salt	Cooling to cold	Salty	Softening
Seaweed	Cooling to cold	Salty, slightly sweet	Cools blood heat
Drinks			
Mineral water	Neutral, cooling to cold	Salty, bland	Enriches *yin*

木 Phase: Wood
Organ Network: Liver–Gallbladder

Food	Thermal Nature	Flavor	Effect
Vegetables			
Artichoke	Cooling	Bitter, slightly sweet	Cools liver heat
Eggplant	Cooling	Sweet, slightly bitter	Cools blood and heat
Sauerkraut	Cooling	Sour	Cools heat from intestine and stomach
Spinach	Cooling	Sweet, slightly bitter	Cools liver and blood
Tomato	Cooling to cold	Sweet, sour	Supports liver *yin*
Fruit			
Apple	Neutral to cooling	Slightly sour, sweet,	Stops diarrhea
Apricot	Neutral to warming	Sour, sweet	Supplements body fluids
Currant	Cooling	Sour	Astringent, forms body fluids and blood
Blueberry	Cooling	Sour	Astringent, inhibits diarrhea
Cranberry	Cooling to neutral	Sour	Increases appetite
Gooseberry	Cooling	Sour	Cools heat, cools intestine
Grapefruit	Cooling to cold	Sour	Quenches thirst, downbears *qi*
Kiwi	Cold	Sour, sweet	Cools heat
Lemon	Cold	Very sour	Expels heat
Mango	Cooling	Sour, sweet	Forms body fluids and blood
Orange	Cooling to cold	Sweet, sour	Supplements body fluids
Peach	Neutral to warming	Sour, sweet	Supplements body fluids
Pear	Neutral to cooling	Sweet, slightly sour	Cools stomach heat, moistens
Pineapple	Cooling to neutral	Sweet, sour	Activates digestion
Plum	Neutral to warming	Sour, sweet	Cools liver heat
Raspberry	Cooling	Sour, sweet	Mild laxative, diuretic
Rhubarb	Cold	Sour	Astringent, balances intestine
Strawberry	Cooling	Sweet, sour	Forms body fluids and blood
Tangerine	Cooling	Sour	Supplements body fluids

Food	Thermal Nature	Flavor	Effect
Grains			
Grünkern (dried, unripe spelt kernels)	Cooling	Sweet, slightly sour	Cools liver heat
Rye	Neutral	Sweet, slightly bitter	Strengthens and supplements *qi*
Spelt	Neutral to warming	Sweet	Supplements spleen *qi*
Wheat	Cooling	Sweet	Supplements *qi*, blood, and *yin*
Wheat bran	Cooling	Sweet	Strengthens center burner
Wheat flour	Neutral to warming	Sweet	Moistens, enriches *yin*
Wheat germ	Cooling to cold	Sweet, slightly acrid	Cools liver heat
Dairy Products			
Cream cheese	Cooling to cold	Slightly sour	Moistening
Sour cream	Neutral to cool	Sour, sweet	Enriches *yin*
Yogurt	Cooling to cold	Sour, sweet	Enriches *yin*, cools intestine
Meat			
Rabbit	Neutral to cooling	Slightly sour	Cools blood
Spices			
Vinegar	Warming	Sour, slightly acrid	Moves *qi*, loosens stagnation, improves circulation, stimulates gastric juices
Herbs			
Peppermint	Cooling	Acrid, slightly sweet	Cools heat, loosens phlegm
Rhubarb root	Cold	Bitter	Astringent for intestine, loosens constipation
Sorrel	Cooling	Sour	Diuretic, cools heat
Wood sorrel (shamrock, oxalis acetosella)	Cooling	Sour	Cools blood heat
Beverages, Alcoholic Beverages			
Beer	Cooling to cold	Bitter, sweet	Cools liver heat
Bread juice	Cooling	Sour	Preserves body fluids
Cider	Cooling	Sour	Cools heat, preserves body fluids
Cider vinegar	Neutral	Sour, slightly acrid	Moves *qi*, loosens stagnation, stimulates appetite
Red wine vinegar	Warming	Sour	Moves *qi*, loosens stagnation, stimulates appetite

Food	Thermal Nature	Flavor	Effect
Sherry vinegar	Warming	Sour	Moves *qi*, stimulates appetite
Tea, black	Neutral	Bitter	Stimulates stomach and intestine
Tea, green	Cooling	Bitter	Supplements heart and liver *yin*
White wine	Cooling	Sour, sweet	Enriches *yin*

火 Phase: Fire
Organ Network: Heart–Small Intestine

Food	Thermal Nature	Flavor	Effect
Vegetables			
Belgian endive hearts	Cooling	Bitter, sweet	Cools liver heat
Dandelion	Cooling to cold	Bitter	Cools liver heat
Fruit			
Elderberry	Cooling to neutral	Bitter, sweet	Balances intestine
Peach	Neutral to warming	Sweet, sour	Supplements body fluids
Watermelon	Cold	Sweet	Cools heat
Grains			
Oats	Neutral to warming	Sweet, slightly bitter	Supplements *qi* and *yang*
Spices			
Cardamom	Warming	Acrid, slightly bitter	Stimulates digestion
Chili pepper	Hot	Acrid	Expels cold
Cinnamon bark	Warming to hot	Acrid	Astringent, expels cold
Cinnamon twigs	Warming	Acrid, bitter	Stimulates digestive organs
Coriander	Neutral to cooling	Bitter, acrid	Stimulates digestion
Cumin	Warming	Bitter, acrid	Dries phlegm–cold
Curry	Warming to hot	Acrid, bitter	Stimulates digestion
Paprika	Mildly warming	Bitter, slightly sweet	Stimulates digestion
Rose paprika (sweet paprika)	Warming	Bitter, acrid	Expels damp–cold
Saffron	Neutral to cooling	Sweet, bitter, acrid	Balances spleen and liver
Turmeric (curcuma)	Warming	Bitter, acrid	Dries phlegm–cold
Herbs			
Basil	Warming	Acrid, bitter, slightly sweet	Stimulates digestion, loosens phlegm
Bitter orange peel	Neutral to cooling	Bitter, slightly acrid, slightly sweet	Stimulates digestion
Dandelion	Cooling to cold	Bitter	Cools liver heat
Linseed	Warming	Sweet, bland	Protects mucous membrane

Food	Thermal Nature	Flavor	Effect
Marjoram	Neutral	Bitter, acrid	Astringent, calms digestion
Rosemary	Warming	Bitter, acrid	Stimulates digestion, antispasmodic
Sage	Warming	Bitter, acrid,	Mild clearing of phlegm–cold
Thyme	Warming	Bitter, acrid	Dries, moves *qi*
Beverages, Alcoholic Beverages			
Grain coffee (from roasted barley, spelt, figs, acorns, etc.)	Neutral	Bitter	Stimulates stomach, liver, and gallbladder
Cocoa	Neutral	Bitter, sweet	Strengthening, stimulating
Coffee	Warming	Bitter	Stimulates heart and circulation
Honey	Neutral	Very sweet	Supplements *qi*, moistens
Liqueur, spirits	Hot	Acrid, bitter, sweet	Dispel internal cold
Red wine	Warming	Bitter, acrid, sweet	Enriches *yang*
Tea, black	Neutral	Bitter	Stimulates stomach and intestine
Tea, green	Cooling	Bitter	Supplements heart and liver *yin*

Foods from A to Z

Food	Thermal Nature	Flavor	Effect
A			
Almond	Neutral	Sweet, slightly bitter	Moistens lung
Alpine wild garlic (allium ursinum)	Neutral to warming	Acrid	Detoxifies, moves *qi*
Angelica	Warming	Acrid, bitter, sweet	Supplements center burner and digestion
Aniseed	Warming	Acrid, sweet	Stimulates digestion
Apple	Neutral to cooling	Sweet, slightly sour	Remedies diarrhea
Apricot	Neutral to warming	Sweet, sour	Supplements body fluids
Arugula (rocket, rucola)	Neutral to cooling	Acrid, bitter	Stimulates appetite
Arnica	Neutral	Bitter, slightly sweet, acrid	Supplements heart *qi* and blood circulation
Artichoke	Cooling	Bitter, slightly sweet	Cools liver heat
Asparagus	Cooling	Sweet, bitter	Supplements lungs, kidney *yin*
B			
Banana	Cold	Sweet	Moistens large intestine
Barley	Cooling	Sweet, slightly salty	Expels heat
Bay leaf (bay laurel)	Warming	Acrid, bitter	Stimulates digestion
Basil	Warming	Acrid, bitter, slightly sweet	Stimulates digestion, loosens phlegm
Bass	Neutral	Sweet, slightly salty	Supplements *qi* and blood
Bean, adzuki	Neutral	Sweet, sour	Balances *qi* and blood, balances *yin* (spleen)
Bean, black	Neutral	Sweet	Supplements spleen and kidneys
Bean, broad (fava bean)	Neutral	Sweet	Supplements spleen, removes dampness
Bean, green	Neutral	Sweet	Supplements blood and *qi*
Bean, white	Neutral to cool	Sweet	Supplements spleen
Beef	Neutral	Sweet	Supplements *qi* and blood
Beer	Cooling to cold	Bitter, sweet	Cools liver heat
Beet	Neutral	Sweet, slightly bitter	Balances spleen and stomach *qi*

Food	Thermal Nature	Flavor	Effect
Belgian endive hearts	Cooling	Bitter, sweet	Cools liver heat
Birch leaf	Cooling	Slightly bitter, acrid	Detoxifies, cools heat
Bell pepper, green	Cooling	Slightly acrid, bitter	Moves *qi* and blood
Bell pepper, orange and red	Neutral	Sweet, slightly acrid, bitter	Strengthens center burner
Bell pepper, green	Cooling	Slightly acrid, bitter	Moves *qi* and blood
Bitter orange peel	Neutral to cooling	Bitter, slightly acrid, slightly sweet	Stimulates digestion
Blackberry	Cooling	Sweet, sour	Astringent, forms body fluids and blood
Blackthorn	Cooling	Sour	Astringent, balances intestine
Blueberry	Cooling	Sweet, sour	Astringent, inhibits diarrhea
Bone marrow	Neutral to warming	Sweet, fatty	Moistens, supplements
Borage	Cooling to cold	Bitter, slightly sweet, salty	Moistens, anti-inflammatory
Brazil nut	Neutral	Sweet, slightly bitter	Strengthens spleen, lung
Bean, broad (fava bean)	Neutral	Sweet	Supplements spleen, removes dampness
Broccoli	Cooling	Sweet, slightly bitter	Cools liver and blood
Bread juice	Cooling	Sour	Retains body fluids
Buckwheat	Cooling	Sweet, slightly bitter	Strengthens spleen, loosens phlegm
Butter	Neutral to cool	Sweet, fatty	Supplements blood, *qi*, moistens
Butterbur root	Warming	Slightly acrid, bitter	Loosens phlegm–cold
Buttermilk	Cooling	Sweet	Moistens, cools heat
C			
Cabbage, green	Neutral to warming	Acrid, sweet	Balances stomach and spleen
Cabbage, red	Neutral to warming	Acrid, sweet	Balances spleen, stomach, blood
Canola oil	Warming	Sweet, fatty	Moistens, laxative
Caraway seed	Warming	Acrid, sweet	Stimulates digestion
Cardamom	Warming	Acrid, slightly bitter	Stimulates digestion

Food	Thermal Nature	Flavor	Effect
Carp	Neutral	Sweet, slightly salty	Supplements *qi* and blood
Carrot	Neutral	Sweet	Supplements center burner
Cashew nut	Neutral	Sweet, fatty	Strengthens stomach and intestine
Cauliflower	Neutral to cool	Sweet, slightly bitter	Cools lungs, stomach heat
Caviar	Cold	Salty	Supplements kidney *yin*
Cayenne pepper	Hot	Very acrid	Expels cold
Celery root (celeriac)	Cooling	Sweet, slightly bitter	Cools stomach heat and liver heat
Celery (stalk)	Cooling	Slightly salty and bitter	Cools stomach and liver heat, loosens *qi* stagnation
Chamomile	Neutral	Slightly bitter, sweet	Harmonizes digestion
Chard	Cooling	Sweet, bitter	Cools lung heat
Cheese, cow's milk	Neutral to warming	Sweet, sour	Moistens, warming
Cheese, goat's milk	Warming	Acrid, salty, moderately sweet	Warming
Cheese, sheep's milk	Warming	Acrid, salty, moderately sweet	Warming
Cherry	Warming	Sweet	Nourishes blood
Chervil	Cooling to neutral	Bitter, slightly sweet	Cools blood heat
Chestnut	Warming	Sweet	Strengthens spleen and kidneys
Chicken	Warming	Sweet	Supplements blood and *qi*
Chicken egg	Neutral	Sweet	Supplements blood and *yin*
Chickpea (garbanzo)	Neutral	Sweet	Strengthens spleen *qi* and kidneys
Chili pepper	Hot	Acrid	Expels cold
Chinese (napa) cabbage	Neutral to cooling	Sweet	Cools heat, diuretic
Chinese leek (garlic chives)	Warming	Acrid	Moves *qi*, strengthens center burner
Chives	Warming	Acrid, slightly bitter	Stimulates digestion
Cider	Cooling	Sour	Cools heat, preserves body fluids
Cider vinegar	Neutral	Sour, slightly acrid	Stimulates appetite

Food	Thermal Nature	Flavor	Effect
Cinnamon bark	Warming to hot	Acrid	Astringent, expels cold, diarrhea remedy
Cinnamon twig	Warming	Acrid, bitter	Stimulates digestive organs
Clove	Warming	Acrid	Expels damp cold
Cocoa	Neutral	Bitter, sweet	Strengthening, stimulating
Coconut	Cooling	Sweet	Clears heat
Coconut oil	Cooling	Sweet, fatty	Moistening
Coffee	Warming	Bitter	Stimulates heart *yang*
Coriander	Neutral to cooling	Bitter, acrid	Stimulates digestion
Corn	Neutral to warming	Sweet	Supplements *qi* and blood
Corn silk	Cooling	Slightly sweet	Astringent, clears damp–heat
Cottage cheese	Cooling to cold	Sweet, slightly sour	Moistening
Crab (sweet water)	Cold	Sweet	Enriches *yin*
Cranberry	Cooling to neutral	Sweet, sour	Increases appetite
Crayfish	Cold	Sweet	Enriches *yin*
Cream	Neutral	Sweet, fatty	Supplements *qi* and blood, moistens
Cream cheese	Cooling	Sweet	Moistens, cools heat
Cress, garden	Cooling	Acrid	Balances *qi* and blood
Cucumber	Cold	Sweet, slightly bitter	Cools heat, diuretic
Cumin	Warming	Acrid, sweet	Stimulates digestion, warms center burner
Currant, red	Cooling	Sweet, sour	Astringent, forms body fluids and blood
Curry	Warming to hot	Acrid, bitter	Stimulates digestion
D			
Dandelion	Cooling to cold	Bitter	Cools liver heat
Date	Neutral	Sweet	Supplements blood and body fluids
Dill	Warming	Acrid, slightly bitter	Stimulates appetite
Duck	Neutral to cooling	Sweet, slightly salty	Supplements *qi*, blood, and *yin*
E			
Eel	Warming	Sweet, fatty	Supplements *qi* and blood
Eggplant	Cooling	Sweet, slightly bitter	Cools blood and cools heat

Food	Thermal Nature	Flavor	Effect
Elderberry	Cooling to neutral	Bitter, sweet	Balances intestine
Elderberry flowers	Neutral to cooling	Bitter, sweet, slightly acrid	Expels damp–heat from lungs
F			
Fennel (bulb)	Warming	Sweet, acrid	Balances *qi*, harmonizes center burner
Fennel seed	Warming	Acrid, sweet	Stimulates digestion
Fenugreek seed	Warming	Very bitter, acrid	Loosens phlegm, strengthens
Fig (fresh)	Neutral to warming	Sweet	Strengthens center burner, moistens
Flax seed (linseed)	Warming	Sweet, bland	Protects mucous membrane
Fumaria	Cooling	Bitter, slightly salty	Loosens liver *qi* stagnation
G			
Garlic	Warming to hot	Acrid	Moves *qi*, loosens phlegm
Ghee	Neutral	Sweet, fatty	Supplements blood and *qi*, moistens
Ginger	Warming to hot	Acrid, slightly sweet	Loosens phlegm–cold
Goat meat	Warming	Sweet	Supplements spleen *yang* and kidney *yang*
Goldenrod	Cooling	Bitter	Astringent, expels damp–heat from bladder
Goose	Neutral	Sweet	Supplements spleen *qi*
Gooseberry	Cooling	Sweet, sour	Cools heat, cools intestine
Grain coffee (from roasted barley, spelt, chicory root, figs, acorns, etc.)	Neutral	Bitter	Stimulates stomach, liver and gallbladder
Grape	Neutral to warming	Sweet	Supplements blood and *qi*
Grapefruit	Cooling to cold	Sweet, sour	Quenches thirst, downbears *qi*
Green bean	Neutral	Sweet	Strengthens *qi* and blood
Green (spring) onion	Warming	Acrid	Opens stomach and lungs
Grünkern (dried, unripe spelt kernels)	Cooling	Sweet, slightly sour	Cools liver heat

Food	Thermal Nature	Flavor	Effect
H			
Hazelnut	Neutral to warming	Sweet, fatty	Supplements spleen and kidneys
Herring	Neutral cooling	Sweet, slightly salty	Supplements blood and *qi*
Honey	Neutral	Sweet	Supplements *qi* and blood
Horseradish	Warming, heating	Very acrid	Enriches *yang*, expels wind–cold
Horsetail	Cold	Slightly bitter, bland	Astringent, expels heat, dries dampness
I			
Iceland moss (lichen)	Cooling	Bitter, slightly sweet	Enriches *yin*, relieves cough
Irish moss (carrageen; a seaweed)	Cooling	Slightly sweet, salty, insipid	Enriches *yin*, cools blood heat
J			
Jasmine blossoms	Warming	Acrid, slightly sweet	Supplements lower burner
Juniper berry	Warming	Slightly acrid, bitter	Diuretic
K			
Kale	Neutral to warming	Acrid, sweet	Balances stomach and spleen
Kiwi	Cold	Sweet, sour	Cools heat
Kohlrabi	Neutral	Acrid, sweet	Supplements liver, gallbladder and kidneys
L			
Lady's mantle	Cooling to cold	Slightly bitter	Astringent, cools blood heat
Lamb	Warming to hot	Sweet, slightly bitter	Supplements kidney and spleen *yang*
Lard, pork	Neutral to cooling	Sweet, fatty	Moistens
Lavender	Cooling	Slightly bitter, acrid	Calming, analgesic
Leek	Warming	Acrid, sweet	Moves *qi*, warms Center burner
Lemon	Cold	Very sour	Expels heat
Lemon zest	Cooling	Bitter, slightly acrid	Expels heat, phlegm and toxins
Lentil, green	Neutral	Sweet	Supplements *qi* and blood
Lentil, red	Neutral to warming	Sweet	Supplements *qi* of kidneys and heart
Lettuce (e.g., butter and similar types)	Cooling to cold	Sweet, slightly bitter	Cools heat

Food	Thermal Nature	Flavor	Effect
Licorice	Neutral	Very sweet, slightly bitter	Stimulates digestion
Linden flower	Neutral to cooling	Sweet, slightly acrid	Expels wind–heat, calms
Liqueur	Hot	Acrid, bitter, sweet	Expels internal cold
Lobster	Neutral to warming	Sweet, slightly salty	Supplements kidney *qi* and kidney *yang*
Lovage	Cooling	Bitter, acrid	Stimulates digestion
Lychee	Neutral to warming	Sweet, sour	Supplements *qi* and blood
M			
Marjoram	Neutral	Bitter, acrid	Astringent, calms digestion
Mango	Cooling	Sweet, sour	Forms body fluids and blood
Margarine	Neutral	Sweet, fatty	Moistens
Marigold	Neutral	Bitter, sweet, salty, acrid	Expels heat and toxins
Marshmallow	Cooling	Slightly bitter, salty, slightly acrid	Loosens phlegm, softens
Melon	Cooling	Sweet	Cools heat
Milk, cow's	Neutral to cooling	Sweet	Moistens, cools
Milk, goat's	Neutral to warming	Sweet	Supplements spleen *yang* and kidney *yang*
Milk, sheep's	Neutral to warming	Sweet	Moistens, warming
Milk thistle	Warming	Acrid, bitter	Stimulates liver and gallbladder
Millet	Neutral to warming	Sweet, slightly bitter	Supplements *qi* and cools heat
Mineral water	Neutral, cooling to cold	Salty, bland	Enriches *yin* (kidneys)
Mirabelle (small, yellow plum)	Cooling	Sweet, sour	Cools heat
Miso	Neutral to cooling	Salty, slightly sour	Stimulates digestion
Motherwort	Cooling	Bitter, slightly acrid	Supplements heart *qi*, expels heat
Mugwort	Warming	Very bitter, slightly acrid	Stimulates liver and stomach *qi*
Mushroom, button or crimini/portobella	Cooling	Sweet	Cools blood and heat

Food	Thermal Nature	Flavor	Effect
Mussel	Warming	Salty	Supplements liver and kidney *qi* and *yang*
Mustard (prepared)	Warming	Acrid, bitter	Stimulates digestion, lipolysis (digestion of fats)
Mustard seeds	Warming	Acrid	Expels damp cold
N			
Nutmeg	Warming	Acrid	Astringent, expels damp cold
O			
Oats	Neutral to warming	Sweet, slightly bitter	Supplement nerves and *qi*
Octopus (squid)	Neutral to cooling	Sweet, salty	Supplements *qi*, blood and *yin*
Olive oil	Cooling	Sweet, fatty	Moistens, anti-inflammatory
Onion	Warming	Acrid, sweet	Moves *qi*, loosens phlegm
Orange	Cooling to cold	Sweet, sour	Supplements body fluids
Orange blossom	Neutral	Bitter, sweet, slightly acrid	Calms, insomnia remedy
Oregano	Neutral	Slightly acrid, bitter	Stimulates digestion
Oyster	Neutral to cooling	Sweet, salty	Supplements liver, kidneys, blood and *yin*
P			
Papaya	Neutral	Sweet, slightly bitter	Balances stomach *qi*
Paprika, mild	Warming	Bitter, slightly sweet	Stimulates digestion
Parsley leaf	Warming	Slightly acrid, bitter	Stimulates digestion, diuretic
Parsley root	Neutral	Sweet, bland, slightly acrid	Diuretic, supplements kidney *yin*
Parsnip	Neutral to warming	Sweet, bitter, acrid	Balances stomach, intestine, lung
Passion fruit	Cooling	Slightly bitter, bland	Calms, supplements heart *yin*
Peach	Neutral to warming	Sweet, sour	Supplements body fluids
Peanut	Neutral to warming	Sweet, fatty	Moistens lungs
Peanut butter	Neutral	Sweet, fatty	Moistens
Peanut oil	Neutral	Sweet, fatty	Moistens
Pear	Cooling	Sweet, slightly sour	Cools stomach heat

Food	Thermal Nature	Flavor	Effect
Pea, green	Neutral to slightly cool	Sweet	Supplements spleen
Pea, yellow	Neutral	Sweet	Supplements spleen
Pepper, black (ripe; seasoning, not bell pepper)	Warming to hot	Very acrid	Enriches *yang*, expels cold
Pepper, green (unripe; seasoning, not bell pepper)	Warming	Acrid	Enriches *yang*, stimulates *qi* coursing
Pepper, white (fully ripe; seasoning, not bell pepper)	Warming to hot	Very acrid	Enriches *yang*, expels cold
Peppermint	Cooling	Acrid, slightly sweet	Downbears heat, loosens phlegm
Pheasant	Warming	Sweet, slightly sour	Supplements center burner
Pineapple	Cooling to neutral	Sweet, sour	Activates digestion
Pistachio	Neutral	Sweet, slightly bitter	Moistens lung and skin
Plantain (ribwort)	Cold	Bitter	Mildly astringent, anti-inflammatory
Plum	Neutral to warming	Sweet, sour	Cools liver heat
Pollen, bee	Neutral	Sweet–acrid, bitter	Supplements heart
Pork	Cooling	Sweet, fatty	Supplements blood and *yin*
Potato	Neutral	Sweet	Strengthens spleen, supplements *qi* and heals inflammation
Prawn	Warming	Sweet, slightly salty	Supplements kidney *qi* and kidney *yang*
Primrose	Neutral	Slightly sweet, acrid	Alleviates pain, rheumatism/arthritis
Pumpkin	Neutral to warming	Sweet	Supplements center burner, strengthens *qi*
Q			
Quail	Neutral	Sweet	Supplements *qi* of center burner
Quince	Neutral to cooling	Slightly bitter	Supplements intestine

Food	Thermal Nature	Flavor	Effect
R			
Rabbit	Neutral to cooling	Sweet	Cools blood
Rabbit, wild	Neutral to cooling	Sweet	Supplements spleen *qi*
Radish	Cooling	Acrid	Loosens blood stasis, blood heat
Radish, icicle or daikon (raw)	Neutral to cool	Acrid	Loosens phlegm in lungs, stomach
Raspberry	**Cooling**	**Sweet, mildly sour**	**Laxative, diuretic**
Raspberry leaf	Cooling	Slightly bitter	Astringent, expels damp–heat
Red clover	Neutral to cooling	Slightly bitter, bland	Expels toxins, damp–heat
Red wine	Warming	Bitter, acrid, sweet	Enriches *yang*
Red wine vinegar	Warming	Sour	Stimulates appetite
Rhubarb	Cold	Sour	Astringent, balances intestine
Rhubarb root	Cold	Bitter	Astringent for intestine, loosens constipation
Rice	Neutral to warming	Sweet	Supplements *qi*, strengthens center burner
Rose paprika	Warming	Bitter, acrid	Expels damp–cold
Rosemary	Warming	Bitter, acrid	Stimulates digestion, antispasmodic
Rye	Neutral to warming	Sweet, slightly bitter	Supplements and strengthens *qi*
S			
Saffron	Neutral to cooling	Sweet, bitter, acrid	Balances liver, spleen
Sage	Warming, slightly hot	Bitter, acrid,	Expels phlegm–cold
Salmon	Cooling	Sweet, slightly salty, fatty	Supplements *qi* and blood
Salsify	Cooling	Sweet, slightly bitter	Balances and cools blood
Salt	Cooling	Salty	Anti-inflammatory, softens
Sardine	Neutral	Sweet, slightly salty	Supplements *qi* and blood
Sauerkraut	Cooling	Sour	Expels heat from intestine and stomach
Savory	Warming	Acrid, bitter, slightly sweet	Stimulates digestion, loosens phlegm

Food	Thermal Nature	Flavor	Effect
Schnapps (high-proof spirit)	Hot	Acrid, bitter, sweet	Expels internal cold
Sea snail (conch)	Neutral	Sweet, salty	Supplements liver *qi* and *yang* and kidney *qi* and *yang*
Seaweed	Cooling to cold	Salty, slightly sweet	Cools blood heat
Sesame, black	Neutral	Sweet, fatty	Strengthens liver and kidneys
Sesame, white	Cooling	Sweet, fatty	Supplements blood and body fluids
Sesame oil	Neutral to cooling	Sweet, fatty	Moistens skin and intestine
Shark	Neutral	Sweet, slightly salty	Supplements *qi*, blood and *yin*
Shepherd's purse	Cooling	Slightly bitter	Astringent, supplements blood, clears heat
Sherry vinegar	Warming	Sour	Moves *qi*, stimulates appetite
Shrimp	Cold	Sweet, slightly salty	Enriches *yin*
Soft drinks, sodas (artificial)	Cooling to cold	Very sweet	Exhaust center burner
Sorrel	Cooling	Sour	Diuretic, cools heat
Sour cream	Neutral to cooling	Sour, sweet	Nourishes *yin*
Soybean oil	Neutral to warming	Sweet, fatty	Moistens, laxative
Soybean, black	Neutral	Sweet	Supplements spleen and kidneys
Soybean, green	Neutral to cold	Sweet	Expels heat
Soybean, yellow	Neutral to cooling	Slightly sweet	Expels heat
Soybean oil	Neutral to warming	Sweet, fatty	Moistens, laxative
Spelt	Neutral to warming	Sweet	Supplements spleen *qi*
Spinach	Cooling	Sweet, slightly bitter	Cools liver and blood
St. John's wort	Neutral to cooling	Slightly bitter, sweet	Anti-inflammatory
Star fruit	Cooling to cold	Sweet, sour	Cools heat
Stinging nettle	Warming	Bitter, acrid, slightly salty	Balances blood, diuretic
Strawberry	Cooling	Sweet, sour	Forms body fluids and blood
Sunflower oil	Neutral to cooling	Sweet, fatty	Moistens, enriches *yin*
Sunflower seed	Neutral	Sweet, fatty	Nourishes *yin*, moistens
Sweet potato	Neutral to warming	Sweet	Supplements center burner, *qi* and blood

Food	Thermal Nature	Flavor	Effect
T			
Tangerine	Cooling	Sweet, sour	Cools heat, supplements body fluids
Tarragon	Warming	Bitter, slightly acrid	Stimulates digestion
Tea, black	Neutral	Bitter	Stimulates stomach and intestine
Tea, green	Cooling	Bitter	Cools heat and liver *yin*
Thyme	Warming	Bitter, acrid	Extremely drying, stimulates
Tofu	Neutral	Sweet	Expels heat, moistens
Tomato	Cooling to cold	Sweet, sour	Supports liver and *yin*
Trout	Neutral to warming	Sweet	Supplements center burner
Tuna	Neutral to warming	Sweet, slightly salty	Supplements *qi* and blood
Turkey	Warming	Sweet	Supplements *qi* and *yang*
Turmeric (curcuma)	Warming	Bitter, acrid	Dries phlegm– cold
V			
Valerian	Neutral to cooling	Bitter, slightly sweet	Supplements heart *qi*, relaxes
Vanilla	Warming	Sweet	Mildly stimulates spleen and pancreas
Veal	Neutral	Sweet	Supplements spleen *qi*
Venison, red deer, blacktailed deer	Warming	Sweet	Supplements *qi*, blood and *yang*
Venison, reindeer, moose, elk, roe deer	Neutral to warming	Sweet	Supplements *qi* and blood
Verbena	Neutral to cooling	Bitter, slightly acrid	Expels wind–heat
Vinegar	Warming	Sour	Stimulates circulation, gastric juices
W			
Walnut	Warming	Sweet, bitter, fatty	Strengthens kidneys and lung
Walnut oil	Warming	Sweet, fatty	Supplements kidney *yang*
Watercress	Neutral	Acrid, slightly bitter	Stimulates digestion
Watermelon	Cold	Sweet	Cools heat
Wheat bran	Cooling	Sweet	Strengthens center burner
Wheat flour	Neutral to warming	Sweet	Moistens, enriches *yin*

Food	Thermal Nature	Flavor	Effect
Wheat germ	Cooling to cold	Sweet, slightly acrid	Cools liver heat
Wheat germ oil	Cooling	Sweet, fatty	Supplements kidney *yin*
White wine	Cooling	Sour, sweet	Enriches *yin*
Wild boar (pig)	Neutral to warming	Sweet	Supplements *qi* and *yang*
Wood sorrel (shamrock, oxalis acetosella)	Cooling	Sour	Cools blood heat
Y			
Yeast	Refreshing	Sour, sweet, bitter	Stimulates digestion
Yogurt	Cooling to cold	Sweet, sour	Enriches *yin*, cools intestine
Z			
Zucchini	Cooling	Sweet, bitter	Cools stomach and liver heat

7 Glossary

The English and Chinese terminology used in this book is based on "A Practical Dictionary of Chinese Medicine" by Nigel Wiseman and Feng Ye (Paradigm Publications, 1998, 2nd edition). As a quick reference, the following glossary provides a list of some of the most common terms used in this book and their Chinese equivalent, as derived from Nigel Wiseman/Feng Ye.

English Terms	Chinese Terms
Acquired constitution *jing*	*hou tian zhi jing*
Ancestral *qi* (synonym: air *qi* or gathering *qi*)	*zong qi*
Body fluids See also humors, liquids (accordning to Wiseman/Feng *jin* are the thinner fluids, and *ye* are the thicker, turbid ones). Both elements are also partly responsible for blood quality and quantity.	*jin ye*
Bowels and viscera	*zang fu*
Center burner (→Triple burner)	*zhong jiao*
Center *qi*	*zhong qi*
Channel *qi* (synonym: essential *qi*, or vessel *qi*)	*jing qi*
Clear (food or liquid)	*qing*
Cold Impediment	*han bi*
Congenital (constitution) *jing* (synonym: prenatal, inherited *jing*)	*xian tian zhi jing*
Construction *qi*	*yin qi*
Controller Vessel	*ren mai*
Corporeal soul	*po*
Counterflow *qi* (synonym: rebellious or reverse)	*qi ni*
Damp impediment	*shi bi*
Defense *qi*	*wei qi*
Downbear (verb), downbearing (adj.): To descend or cause to descend	*jiang*
Drum distention (synonym: for abdominal distention)	*gu zhang*
Dryness	*zao*
Engendering cycle (synonym: feeding cycle)	*xiang sheng*
Enriching/supplementing *yin*	*zi yin*
Essence (synonym: essential *qi*) Congenital constitution *jing* and acquired constitution *jing*	*jing*
Ethereal soul	*hun*
Extraordinary vessels	*qi jing ba mai*
Fire flaming upward	*huo shang yan*
Five flavors (acridity, sourness, sweetness, bitterness, saltiness)	*wu wei*
Five hearts, or hot areas (soles of feet, palms, inside sternum)	*wu yi*
Five Impediments	*wu bi*

Five minds	*wu shi*
Five phases	*wu xing*
Governing Vessel (GV)	*du mai*
Greater *yang*	*tai yang*
Gu qi (synonym: drum *qi*, bone *qi*, or food *qi*)	*gu qi*
Heat impediment	*re bi*
Humors Turbid, heavy, denser element; moistens and nourishes brain, bone marrow, and lubricates joints. Sweat, snivel, tears, drool, and spittle.	*ve*
Jing (see p. 10)	*jing*
Lesser *yang*	*shao yang*
Liquids Clear, light, thin element; circulates mostly on body surface; keeps skin, hair, ears, eyes, mouth, nose, genitals, and other orifices and muscles moist.	*jin*
Lower burner	*xia jiao*
Mind, willpower	*zhi*
Night sweating (synonym: thief sweating)	*dao han*
Nontransformation of food	*wan gu bu hua*
Original *qi*	*yuan qi*
Overwhelming cycle	*xiang cheng*
Pulse	*mai*
Qi: Vital life force (see p. 10)	*qi*
Qi counterflow	*qi ni*
Qi stagnation	*qi zhi*
Qi vacuity	*qi xu*
Qi vomiting (In the original and in some older English books called rebellious *qi*)	*qi ou*
Rebellion cycle	*xiang wu*
Repletion (→ Vacuity)	*shi*
Repletion heat	*shi re*
Restraining cycle	*xiang ke*
Reverting *yin*	*jue yin*
Right or righting *qi*	*zheng qi*
Sheng cycle (upbearing cycle)	*sheng cycle*

Sinew	*jin*
Spirit	*shen*
Spirit and Kidney ("kidney stores mind/spirit/will power")	*shen*
Stomach fire	*wei huo*
Stomach heat	*wei re*
Stomach *yin* vacuity	*wei yin xu*
Supplement: To increase or strengthen *yin*, *yang*, or *qi*	*bu*
Tongue fur	*she tai*
Triple burner: One of the six bowels, consisting of upper, middle, and lower burner	*san jiao*
True *qi*	*zhen qi*
Turbid (as in food and liquid)	*zhuo*
Upbear (*qi*), upbearing (adj.): To ascend, or cause to ascend	*sheng*
Vacuity (and repletion) The term "vacuity" comes from the Chinese "*xu*" (vacuous, empty, lacking, weak). Its opposite is "repletion," which comes from the Chinese "*shi*." Vacuity and repletion can be present in varying degrees, from slight to complete. In Western terms, vacuity may be viewed as a deficit or deficiency. However, vacuity and repletion are not symptom categories, excesses, or deficiencies, but constitutional imbalances perceptible in the topological character of the body (Manaka). Vacuity is the weakness of right *qi* (*zheng qi*), the forces that maintain the health of the body and fight disease. Repletion is strength of evil *qi* (*xie qi*) or accumulation of physiological products within the body such as phlegm–rheum, water–damp, static blood, and stagnant *qi* (Wiseman).	*xu* (and *shi*)
Viscera	*fu*
Wind impediment	*feng bi*
Yang (see p. 7)	*yang*
Yang brightness	*yang ming*
Yang vacuity	*yang xu*
Yin (see p. 7)	*yin*
Yin humor: Essence, body fluids; blood, liquids, blood, humor	*yin ye*
Yin vacuity	*yin xu*

Further Reading

Dai Y-F, Liu C-J. Fruit as Medicine. Kuranda: The Ram Skull Press; 1986.

Enquin Z, et al. Chinese Medicated Diet. Shanghai: Publishing House of Shanghai College; 1988.

Flaws B. Chinese Medical Wines & Elixirs. Boulder, CO: Blue Poppy Press; 1994.

Flaws B. The Book of Jook. Boulder, CO: Blue Poppy Press; 1995.

Flaws B, Wolfe H. Prince Wen Hui's Cook. Brookline, MA: Paradigm Publications; 1983.

Haas E. Staying Healthy with the Seasons. California: Celestial Arts; 1981.

Hammer L. The Patient–Practitioner Relationship in Acupuncture. Stuttgart–New York: Thieme Publishers; 2009.

Hecker H-U, et al. Practice of Acupuncture. Stuttgart–New York: Thieme Publishers; 2005.

Hecker H-U, et al. Microsystems Acupuncture. Stuttgart–New York: Thieme Publishers; 2006.

Hecker H-U, et al. Color Atlas of Acupuncture. 2nd ed. Stuttgart–New York: Thieme Publishers; 2008.

Hempen C-H, Wortman Chow V. Pocket Atlas of Acupuncture. Stuttgart–New York: Thieme Publishers; 2006.

Higdon J. An Evidence-based Approach to Vitamins and Minerals. New York: Thieme Publishers; 2003.

Huan ZY, Rose K. Who Can Ride the Dragon? Brookline, MA: Paradigm Publications; 1999.

Huang Di Nei Jing: The Yellow Emperor's Classic of Medicine. Beijing: Foreign Language Press; 1986.

Jing-Feng C. Eating your Way to Health. Beijing: Foreign Language Press; 1988.

Kaptchuk T. The Web That Has No Weaver. 2nd ed. Columbus, OH: McGraw-Hill; 2000.

Kasper H. Ernährungsmedizin und Diätetik. Munich: Urban & Fischer; 2000.

Kirschbaum B. Atlas of Chinese Tongue Diagnosis. Vista, CA: Eastland Press; 2000.

Lin Z-H. Pocket Atlas of Pulse Diagnosis. Stuttgart–New York: Thieme Publishers; 2008.

Liu J, Peck G (eds). Chinese Dietary Therapy. Edinburgh: Churchill-Livingstone; 1995.

Lu HC. Chinese System of Food Cures. New York: Sterling; 1986.

Lu HC. Chinese Foods for Longevity. New York: Sterling; 1990.

Maciocia G. Foundations of Chinese Medicine: A Comprehensive Text for Acupuncturists and Herbalists. London: Churchill-Livingstone; 1989.

Maciocia G. The Practice of Chinese Medicine. London: Churchill-Livingstone; 1994.

Nan Jing Jiao Shi. Classic of Difficulties. Edited by Nanjing College of Traditional Chinese Medicine, reprint/revised edition. Beijing: People's Health Publishing House; 1979.

O'Connor J, Bensky D. Acupuncture: A Comprehensive Text. Seattle: Eastland Press; 1981.

Pitchford P. Healing with Whole Foods. Berkeley, CA: North Atlantic Books; 1993.

Schnorrenberger C, Schnorrenberger B. Pocket Atlas of Tongue Diagnosis. Stuttgart–New York: Thieme Publishers; 2005.

Shen Jia-Lin et al. Zhongguo shiliao xue (»Chinesische Diätetik«). Shanghai 1987.

Shi Dian-Hang. Zhongyi shiliao yingyang xue [Dietetics and Nutrition in Chinese Medicine]. Beijing 1988.

Sun Simiao. Qian Jin Fang [Valuable prescriptions worth a thousand gold pieces for emergencies], reprint. Beijing 1992.

Unschuld P. Chinese Medicine. Brookline, MA: Paradigm Publications; 1998.

Unschuld P. Huang Di Nei Jing Su Wen: Nature, Knowledge, Imagery in an Ancient Chinese Medical Text. Berkeley, CA: University of California Press; 2003.

Wiseman N, Feng Y. A Practical Dictionary of Chinese Medicine. 2nd ed. Brookline, MA: Paradigm Publications; 1998.

Yang Ji-Zhou. Compendium of Acupuncture (Zhen Jiu Da Cheng), reprint. Beijing: People's Health Publishing House; 1980.

Yang, Shou-Zhong, Ki Jian-yong. Li Dongyuan's Treatise on the Spleen & Stomach. Boulder, CO: Blue Poppy Press; 1993.

Zhang Zhongjing (Shan Han Lun): Discussion on Cold-induced Diseases, reprint. Edited by Nanjing College of Traditional Chinese Medicine,

Shanghanlun Research Group. Shanghai: Shanghai Scientific Publishing House; 1980.

Index

D

E